Discovering the Herbs of the S

DISCOVERING THE HERBS OF SPRING

Seasonal Medicinal Herbs

Caroline Evans MH

2nd Edition

DISCLAIMER

The contents of this book are for informative purposes only.
The information herein is in no way intended to treat or diagnose. Any use of this information is done so completely at your own risk.
It is recommended that you seek advice of a fully qualified health care professional.

This book and the entire series of 'Discovering the Herbs of the Seasons' are copywrite © to Caroline Evans of Heaven on Earth Herbals.®

This book was self published and printed with the use of Amazon

Copywrite © by Caroline Evans, Heaven on Earth Herbals®
First published March 2022
2nd Edition August 2023

All rights reserved.
No part of this book may be reproduced in any form or by any electronic or mechanical means, including information storage or retrieval systems, without prior written permission from the author, except for the use of brief quotations in a book review.

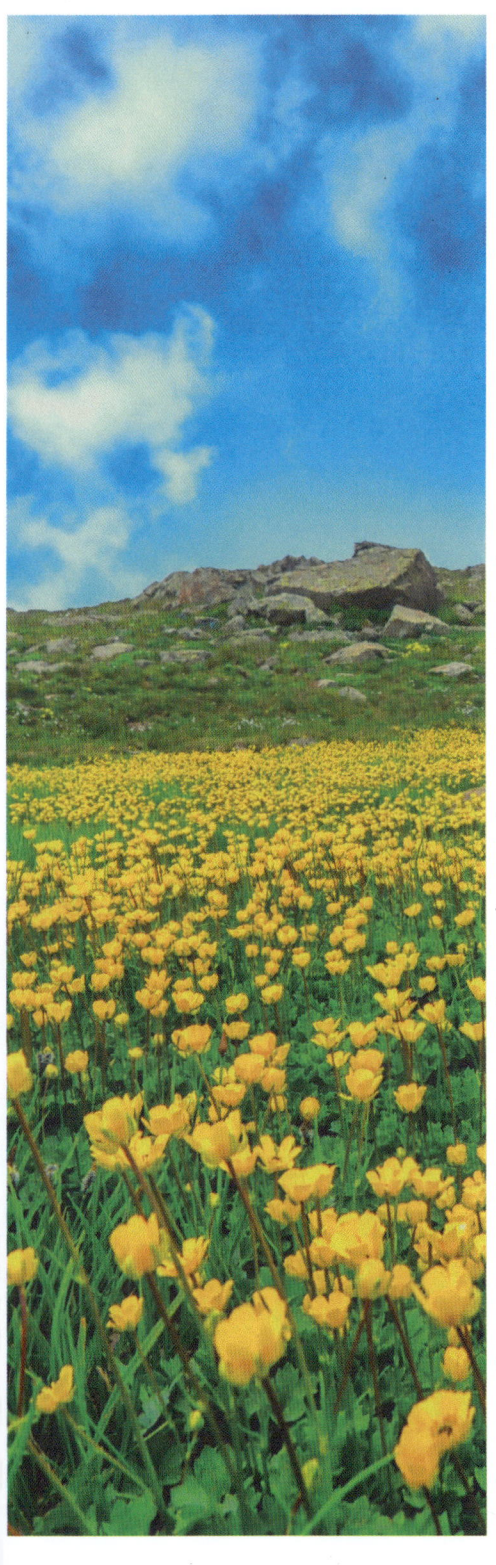

CONTENT
TABLE OF CONTENTS

4 INTRODUCTION

7 GARLIC

15 PRIMROSE

23 DANDELION

33 CLEAVERS

41 CHICKWEED

49 VIOLET

59 PLANTAIN

67 HAWTHORN

76 NETTLE

85 SYMBOLISM

87 GLOSSARY

89 ABOUT THE AUTHOR

AUGUST 2023

INTRODUCTION

We live in an age when it is more important than ever to know:

~ How to feed ourselves

~ How to recognise our local herbs

~ How to make our own medicine

In some small way I hope that this will contribute to your natural autonomy and health freedom.

Remember your health is in your hands!

Alt the best of health & happiness,

Caroline

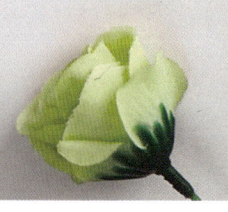

GRATITUDE

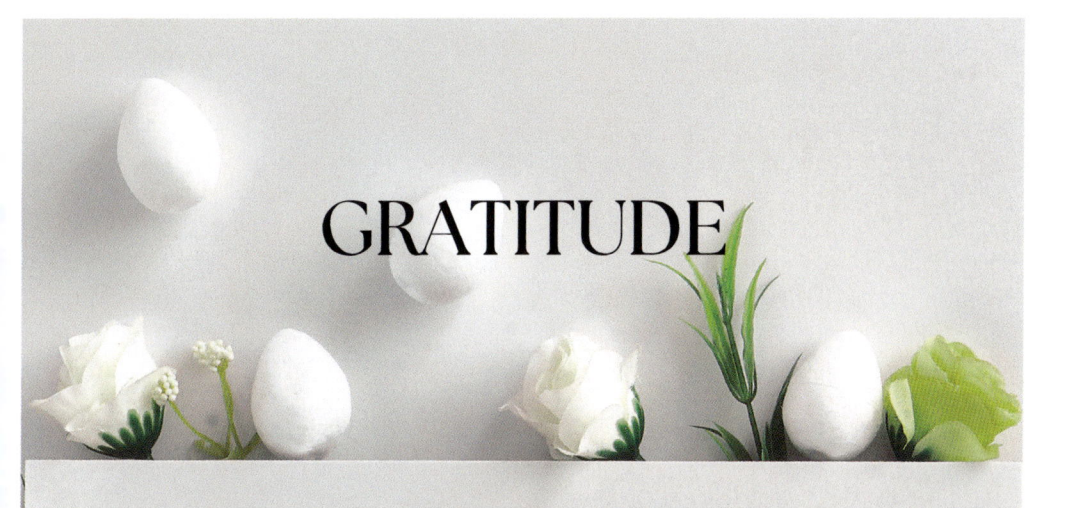

With much love and deep gratitude to my mother Eirys for her continual belief, to Clem for his patience, to my children as my teachers and to all the herbs, flowers and trees that breathe their whispers onto me.

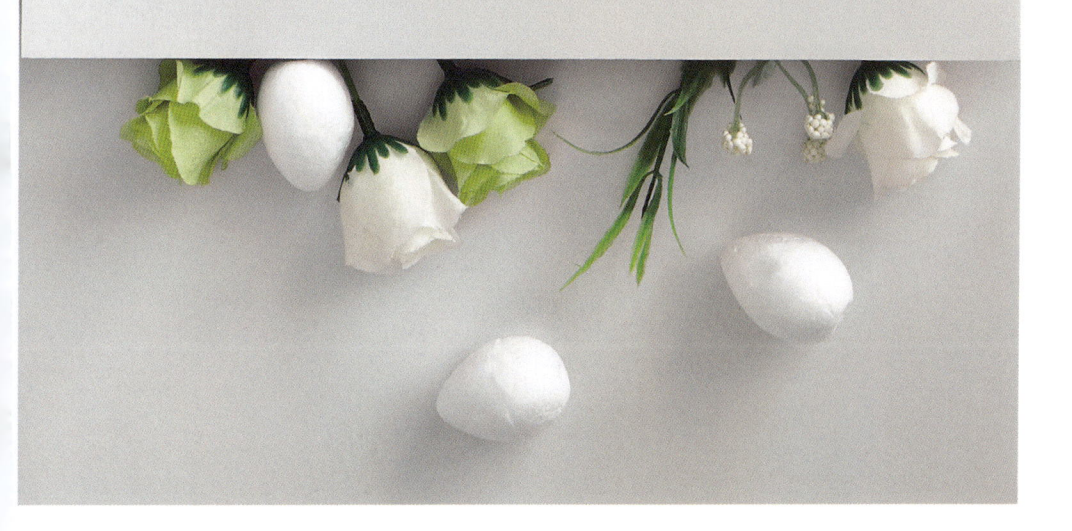

The word 'herb' means 'to heal'

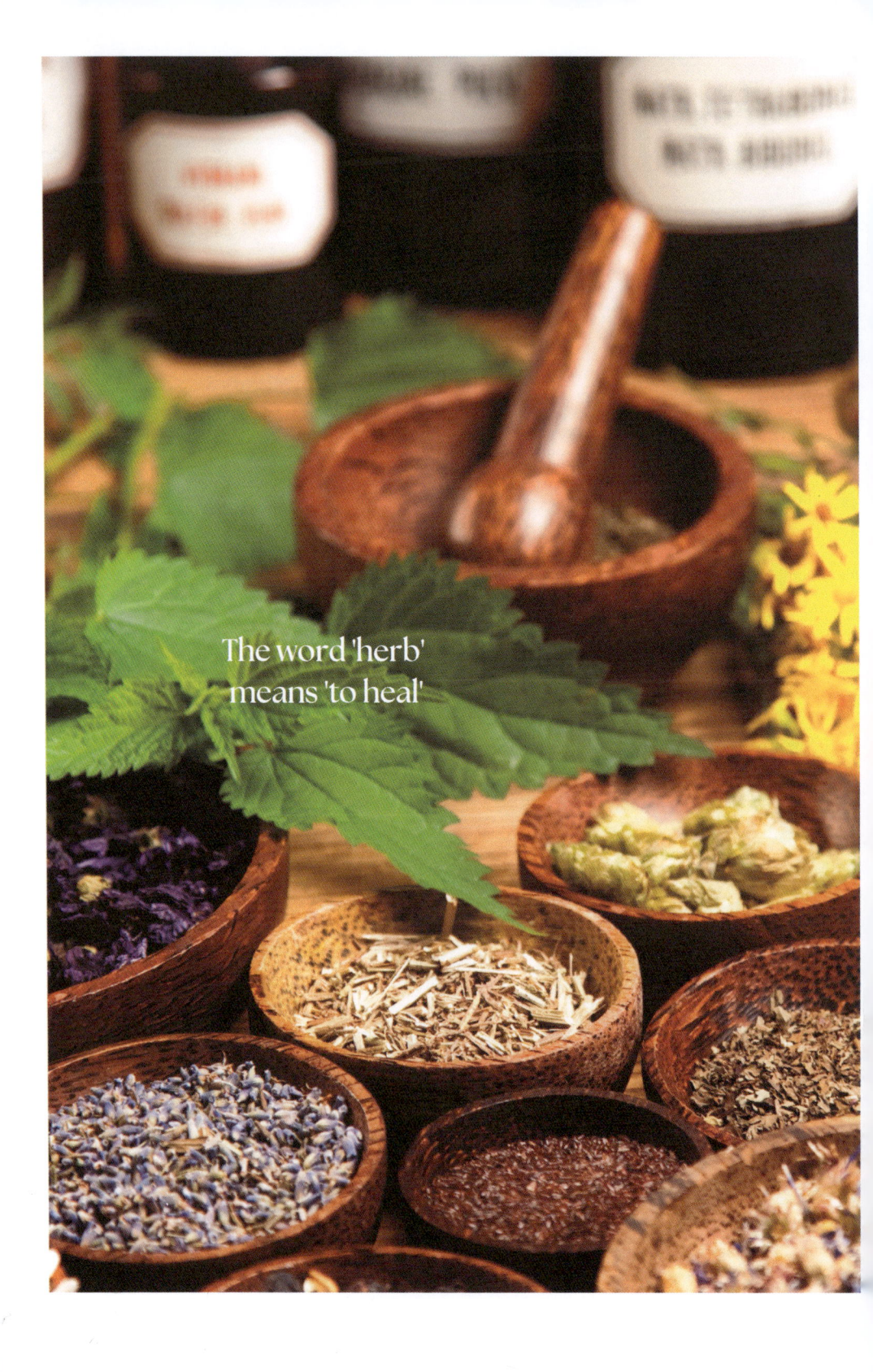

☾ WILD GARLIC

Latin Name: *Allium ursinum*

Family Name: Liliaceae
(Lily, tulip, aloe, onion, leek, garlic, chive)

Other Names: Ramsons, onion garlic, cure-all, Bears garlic

Parts Used: Leaves, Flowers, Buds, stems and green seeds.

Habitat: Ancient wet damp woodlands, and hedgebanks

Identification: The leaf tips appear in earliest Spring and from April, the white star shaped flowers appear.

Looks like Lily of the Valley with hyacinth flowers and Lords and ladies, Cuckoos Pint, with mottled leaves) but the smell is its identifying factor.

Follow your nose!

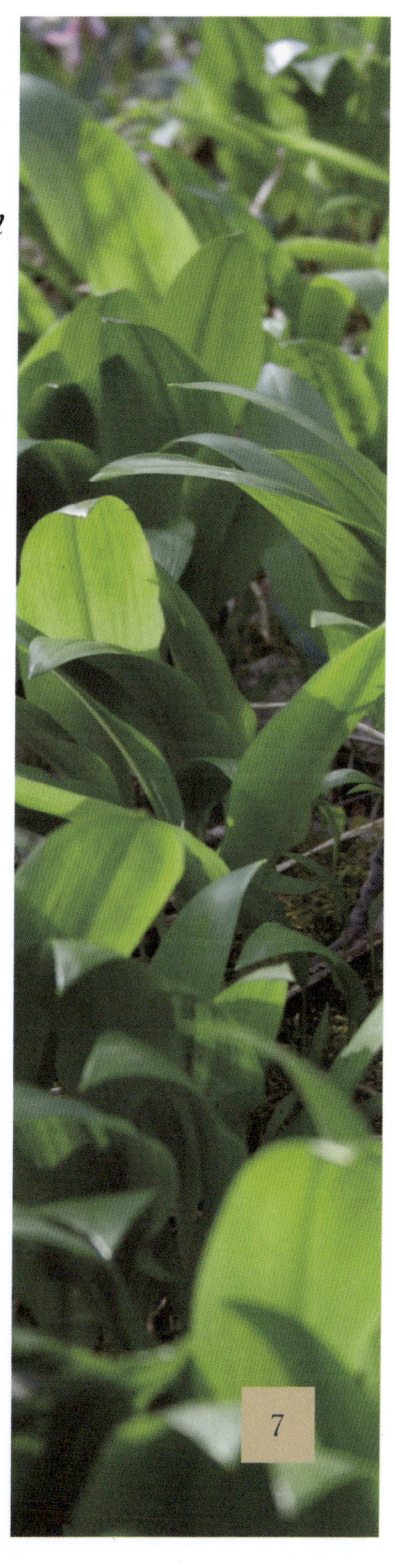

History & Folklore

Garlic dates back 3000 years to the times of the Druids. A herb of our ancestors, finding it in woods indicates you are in ancient woodland.

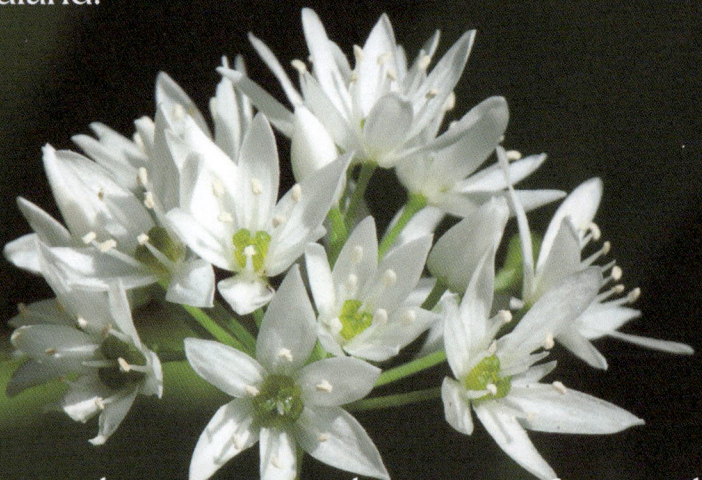

Known as bears garlic as it is a favoured forage of bears who used it to regain their strength after a winters hibernation. The "plants of the bear" are believed to contain the power of renewal and purification. Bulbs were planted as good luck in Irish cottages to ward off fairies. In relation to modern day viruses, in the 1918 Spanish Flu pandemic in Ireland, it was carried in people's pockets to ward off the flu.

Healing Properties

- Antibacterial
- Anti-fungal
- Anti microbial
- Anti-parasitic
- Full of Antioxidants
- Contains Vitamin C
- Antiseptic
- Immune enhancer
- Anti candida
- Prebiotic effects, encourages growth of friendly gut bacteria
- Aids digestion
- Anti carcinogenic
- Detoxification: contains 33 different sulphur compounds to help the liver clear toxins from the body.

Medicinal Uses

Toothache
Warts
Sore throats
Coughs and Colds
Blood purifier
Kidney stones
Liver detoxification
High blood pressure
Rheumatism
Blood Circulation
Cholesterol
Digestive aid
Candida
Immunity

Warning: Do not let cats and dogs ingest this as a compound called n-propyl disulphide can cause them to suffer with serious anaemia.

Recipes With Wild Garlic

PESTO

100gm leaves (and/or stems, flowers, seeds)
50gm parmesan or cheddar cheese finely grated OR
2 tblsp nutritional yeast
50gm toasted pine nuts
2-6 tblsp of olive oil
seasoning to taste

Whizz everything up together in food processor/ nutri bullet, then gently spoon into a jar, and cover with olive oil. It will keep for 2-3 weeks in the fridge or longer canned

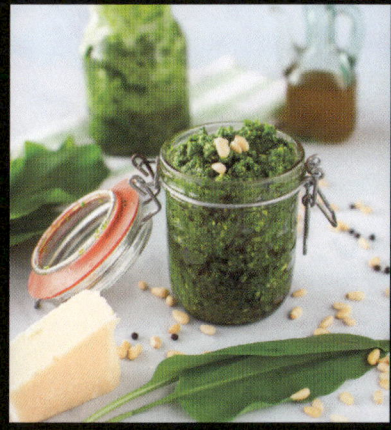

PICKLES

You can pickle any part of wild garlic, the leaves, flowers, buds, seeds or stems. I prefer to use the seeds and flower buds. Just fill a clean jar and cover with vinegar (I use apple cider or white wine vinegar)

Recipes With Wild Garlic

GARLIC SOUP

200gm wild garlic
300gm floury potatoes
1 large onion
seasoning
Cream or coconut cream
olive oil

Chop onion, cook with olive oil for 5 minutes, add chopped garlic leaves, and finally add chopped potatoes, cover with a litre of water or stock. Cook until potatoes start to soften. Whizz up, season, add cream or coconut cream.

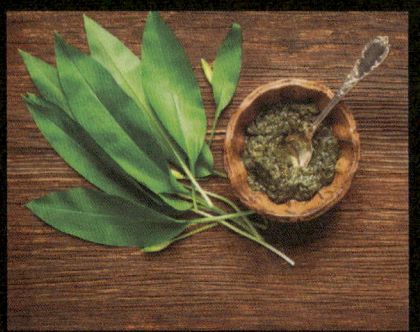

IMMUNITY SYRUP

Fill a jar with flower buds, seeds or leaves and cover with honey a layer and spoon at a time. Leave for a day. Shake well and take 1tsp a day to ward off sickness

COOKING

Wonderful addition to any dish, e.g. omelette, pasta

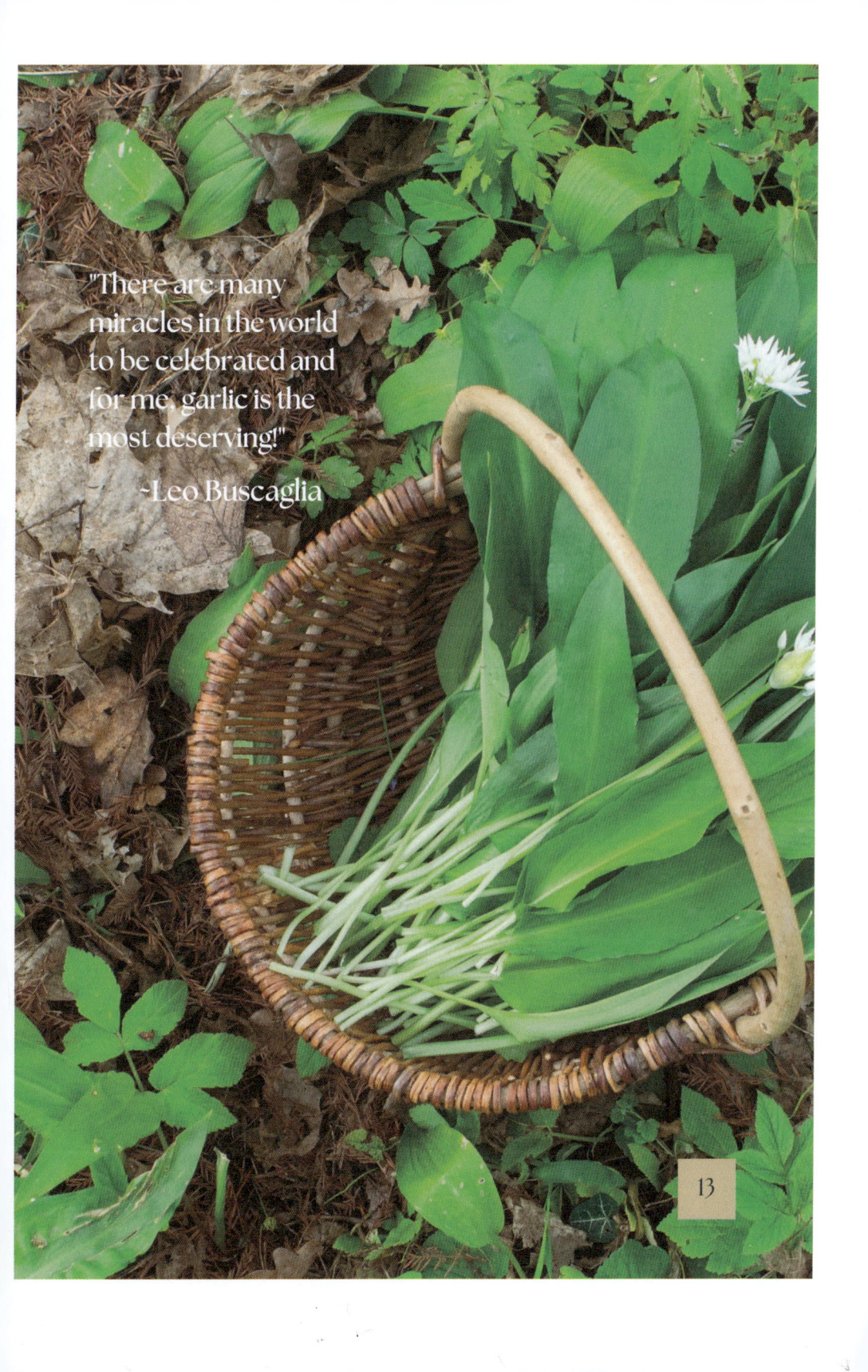

"There are many miracles in the world to be celebrated and for me, garlic is the most deserving!"

~Leo Buscaglia

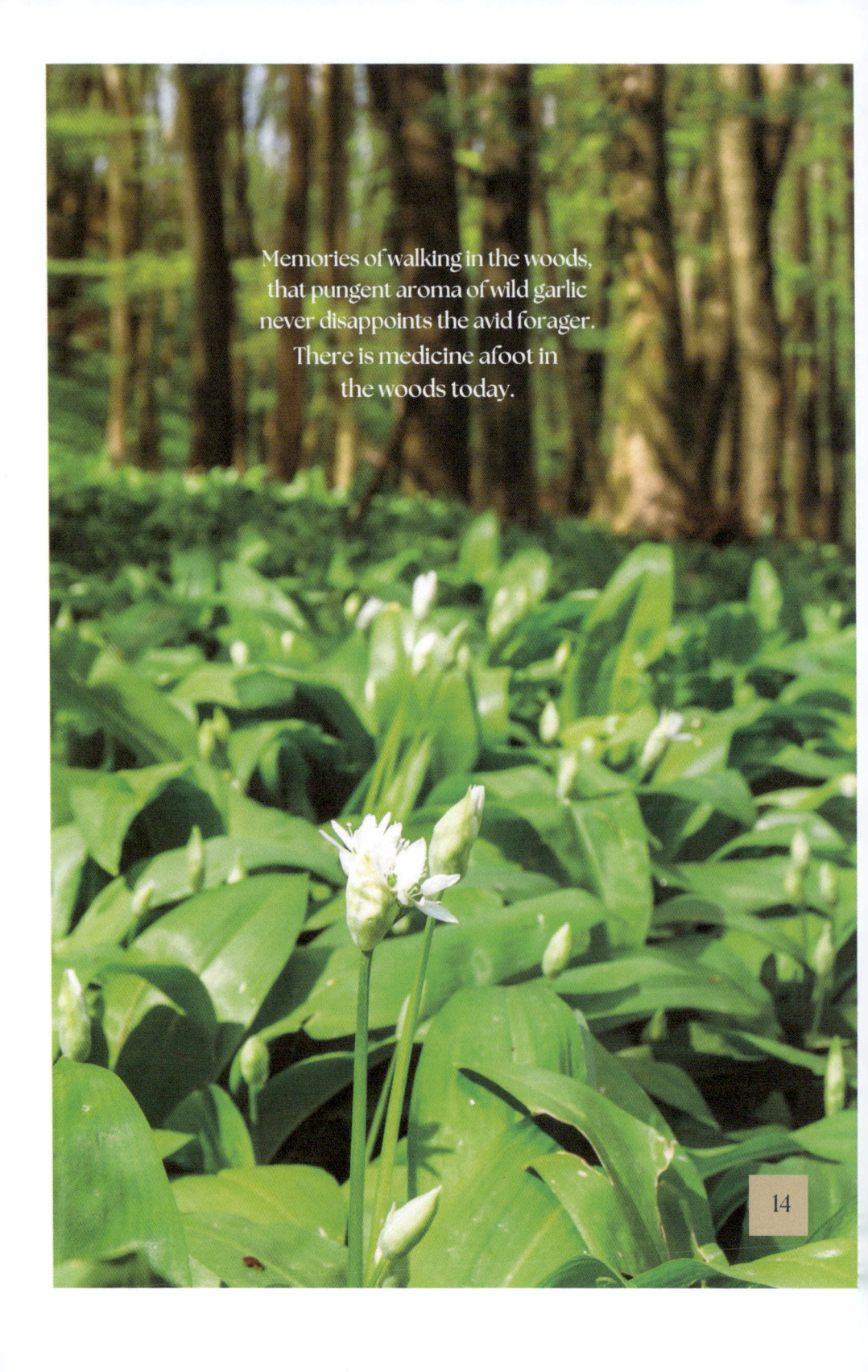

Memories of walking in the woods,
that pungent aroma of wild garlic
never disappoints the avid forager.
There is medicine afoot in
the woods today.

♀ PRIMROSE

Latin Name: *Primula vulgaris*

Family Name: Primulaceae (cowslip, oxlip, scarlet pimpernel, cyclamen)

Other Names: First rose, Fairy cup, English primrose, Butter rose

Parts Used: Petals, flowers

Habitat: One of the first Spring flowers in woods, hedgerows, open pastures, and on lawns. Flowers between February-May.

Identification: The pale yellow petals have deeper yellow centres. The leaves have hairy undersides and wooly stalks. Looks like oxlip, flowers droop to one side and cowslip with bell shaped clustered flowers.

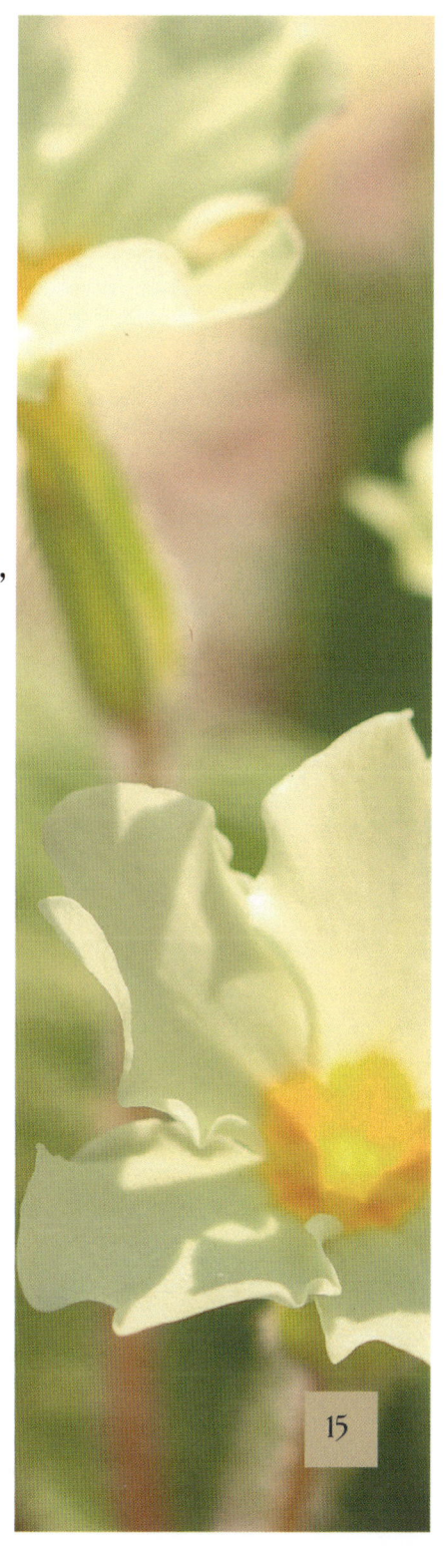

Folklore & History

The term 'primrose' comes from the latin *prima rosa*, which means the first flower. In fact primrose is so famous that she has a whole hill named after her. A major proclamation of a leading druid took place in 1792 and this is what gave Primrose Hill its name because they used primroses in the festival

The Druids believed this was a magical plant, because of its association with the fairies. It is also an important flower for the butterflies.

Nordic mythology associates primrose with the Goddess Freya, Goddess of love, sex and fertility.

Folklore & History

In Celtic folklore it is believed that primroses placed in the doorway protect the home from evil spirits and provide the blessings of the fairies to the home and its inhabitants. They also believed that when one ate primrose flowers they would see the fairies.

It has long been associated with love with and the fairies are said to have used the flowers in love potions so you could give your lover-to-be a cup of primrose tea of the flowers and see what happens, only with their consent of course.

Primrose is considered very magical, symbolising new beginnings and romantic love.

Medicinal Uses

Gout
Rheumatism
Stress
Nervousness
Insomnia
Nervous exhaustion
Headache
Toothache
Depression
Mania
Anxiety
Overwhelm
Neurological issues
Restlessness

NB large doses can induce vomiting

Recipes With Wild Primrose

HERBAL TEA

4-6x fresh flowers or 1 teaspoon of dried flower petals make a cup.

Shake off the flowers when picking to release bugs. Add flowers to a cup, cover with hot water, leave for a few minutes and enjoy.

Add honey to taste if desired. This tea is relaxing, helps when feeling frenzied, anxious, overwhelmed and generally in need of 'calming down'.

HONEY

1/2 cup primrose flowers
200g sugar (I use coconut)
1 pint water

Warm the sugar and water and stir well. Add your primrose flowers and bring gently to the boil. Reduce the heat to a slow simmer and leave to reduce for three hours. The syrup will become a sticky caramel colour, like a darkened honey. Keeps for years.

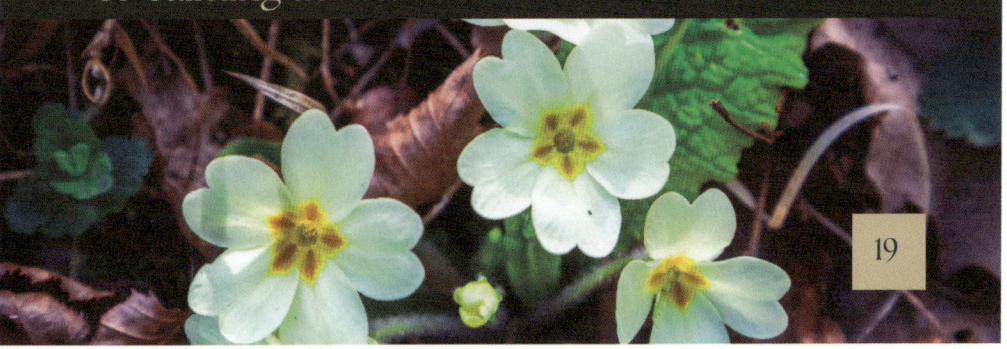

Recipes With Wild Primrose

CANDIED FLOWERS

2x egg whites
Freshly picked primrose flowers set face down to remove bugs
Sugar (i use coconut sugar but they have a browner tinge or xylitol to retain the whiteness but gives a sharp after taste).

Whisk the egg whites together in a bowl. In a second bowl add ground sugar. I tend to grind up coconut sugar in a coffee grinder. Then with a paint-brush, hold the flowers by the stamens and paint egg white on them. Then we carefully dip them into the sugar, shake them off and lay them on some paper or tea towel to dry in a warm dry place.

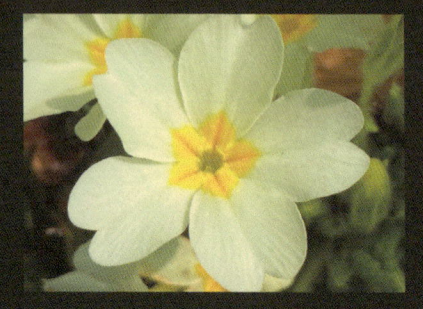

COMPRESS

Bandage a bouquet of primroses onto the heart overnight for anxiety.

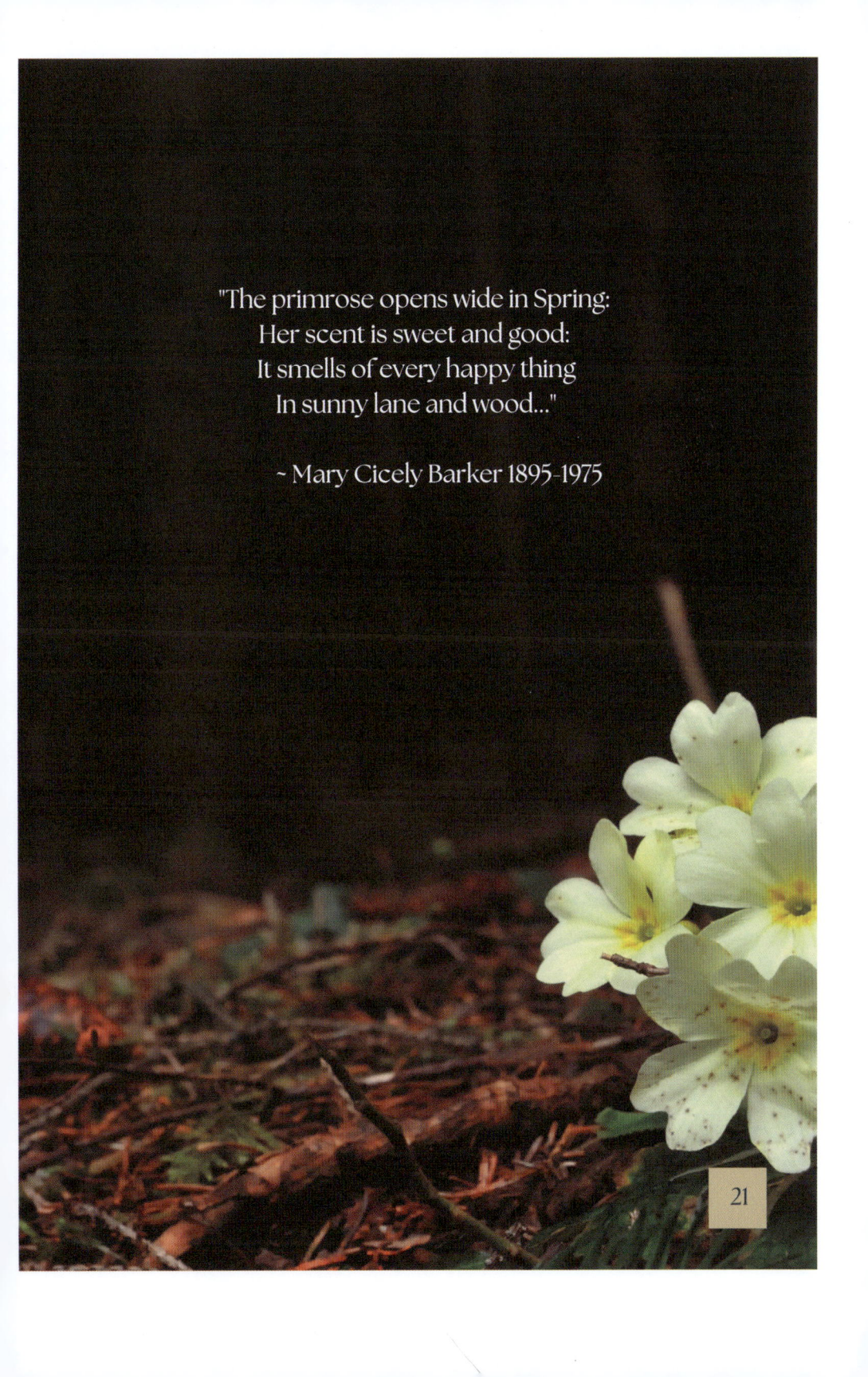

"The primrose opens wide in Spring:
Her scent is sweet and good:
It smells of every happy thing
In sunny lane and wood..."

~ Mary Cicely Barker 1895-1975

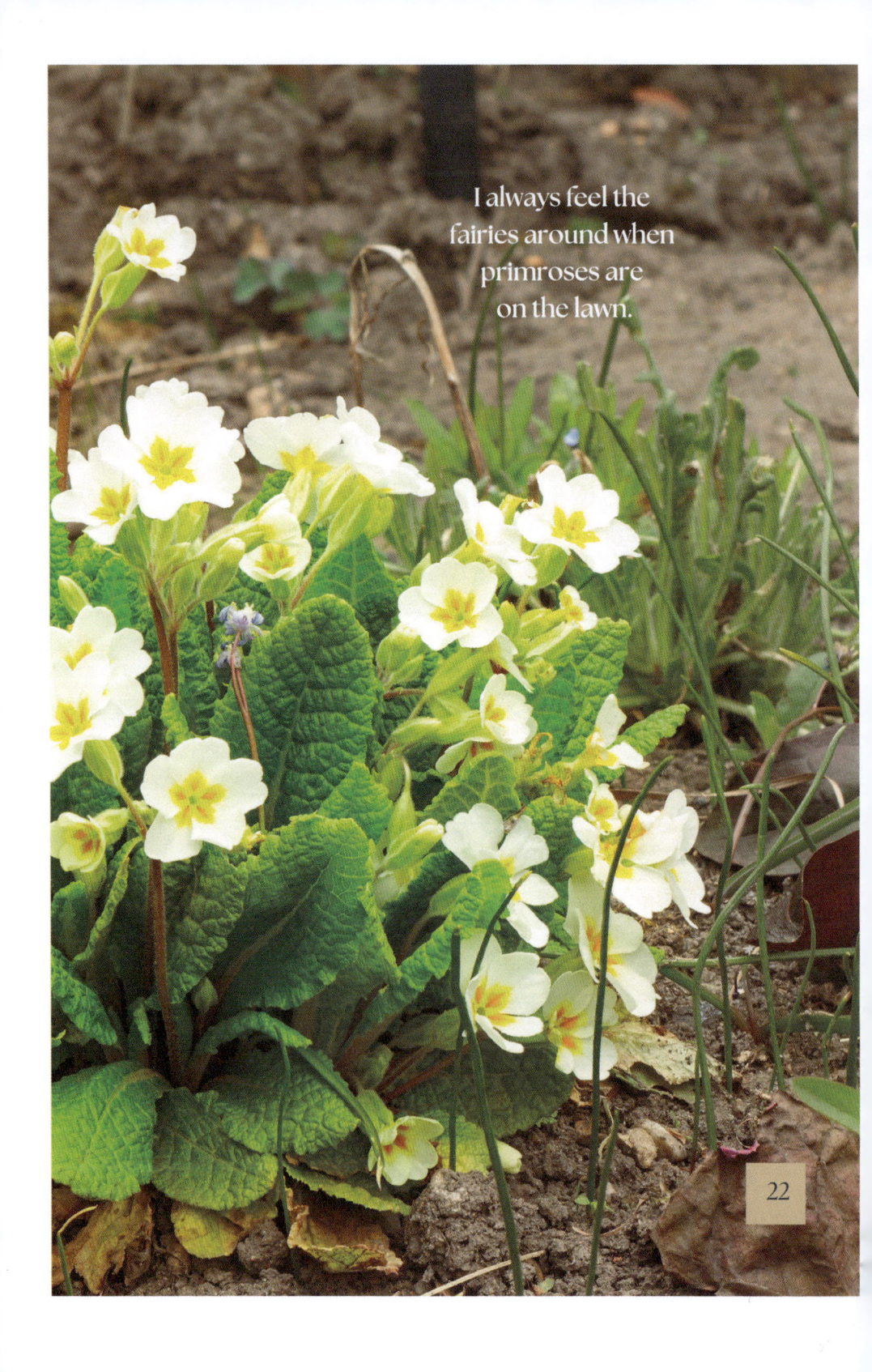

I always feel the
fairies around when
primroses are
on the lawn.

⊙ DANDELION

Latin Name: *Taraxacum officinalis*

Family Name: Asteraceae (Daisy, sunflower, echinacea, calendula, yarrow, chamomile)

Other Names: pis-on-lit, pee-the-bed, dent de lion, lions tooth

Parts Used: Flowers, Leaves, Roots

Habitat: throughout the world at anytime of year growing everywhere even in pavement cracks. Known as a troublesome weed to gardeners however it indicates low calcium levels in the soil.

Identification: Grows to be 2-16 inches high with hollow stems. It exudes a milky substance when cut. Leaves, roughly toothed grow from the base.

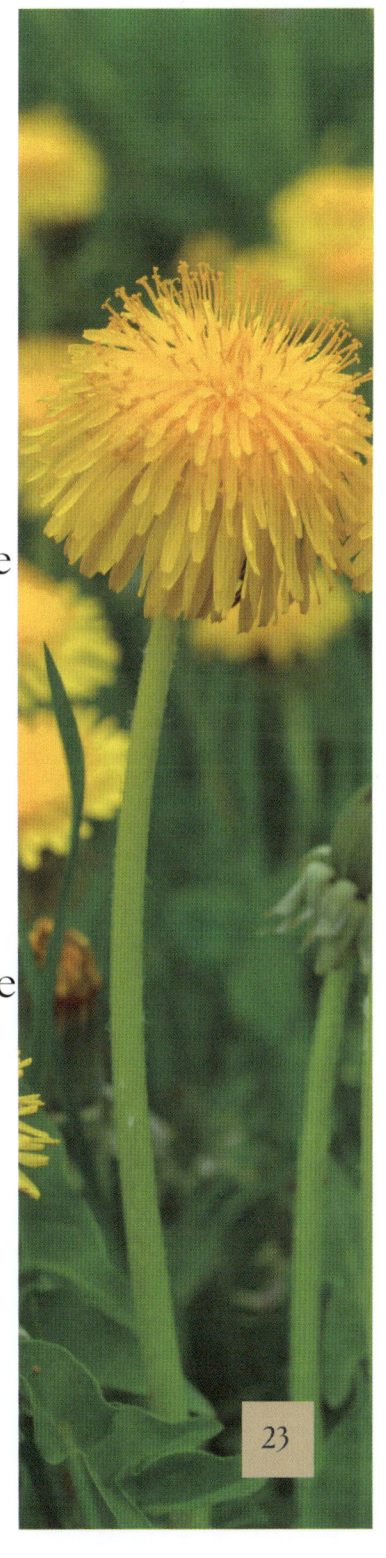

Interesting Fact

The modern gardener will dig up and destroy our humble dandelion. Little realising that the dandelion shows a calcium deficiency in the soil.

Dandelion is packed full of calcium, and will replenish the soil with calcium.

When the dandelion has done its job, it will no longer spring up in your garden. So when we tug at its roots, dandelion gets a signal from Nature to grow some more.

Hence the gardeners trying to rid themselves of this 'weed' would be best to let dandelion grow and fill the soil of calcium first.
Trust in Nature's way.

History & Folklore

The angel of flowers came down to Earth one day to find out who her favourite flower was so she began speaking to each of the flowers. She asked each of the flowers, 'where would each of them like to grow?' First she asked the tulip, "where would you like to grow?' The tulip said, "I would like to grow on a castle lawn with velvety earth beneath me".

She said "you are not my favourite flower. Next she asked the violets, who said, "we want to grow in the woodlands protected from the harsh sunshine. The angel of flowers said "you are not my favourite flower, 'I'm not going to see you"

History & Folklore

So she said to the dandelion "where do you want to grow?" and the dandelion said "I want to grow wherever there are children. I want to grow where the children run past, on their way home from school. I want to grow where there is laughter everywhere".

The angel of flowers said "Do you know what dandelion, you are my absolute favourite, you will grow everywhere, you will have the longest lifespan of any flower, you will grow from Spring to Autumn and you will grow on lawns and hedges and by the sides of the roads" and so it was!

Healing Properties

Diuretic

Hepatic

General Tonic

Anti-rheumatic

Cholagogue

Hepatoprotective

Anti-inflammatory

Antioxidant

Blood purifier

Bitter

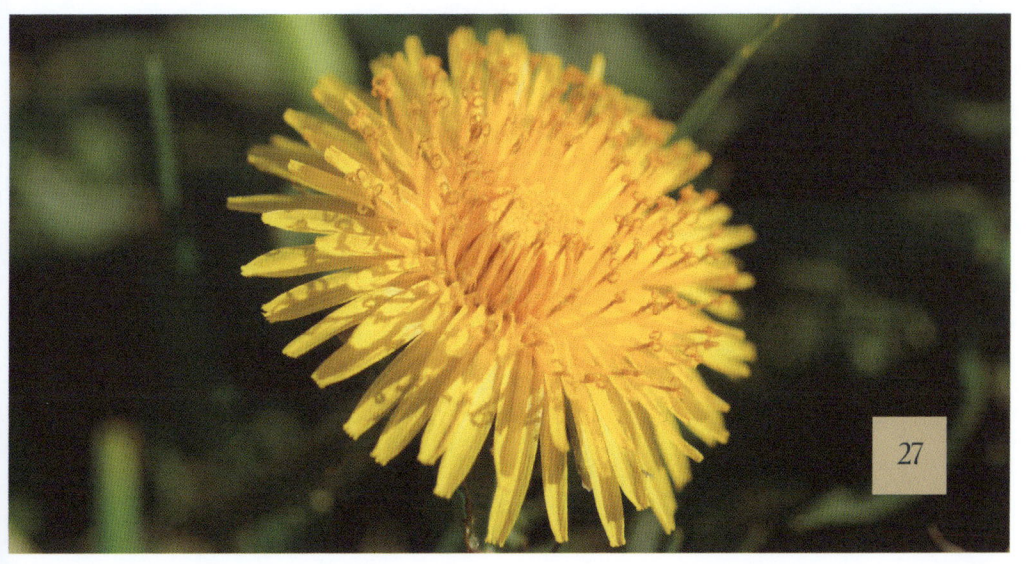

Medicinal Uses

Inflammation of the Gall Bladder
Protects the liver from the effects of coffee and drugs
Liver disorders & Jaundice
Rheumatism and Arthritis
Elevated Cholesterol
Promotes Weight loss
Aids Fat Digestion
Hepatitis C
Indigestion
Kidney disorders
Oedema
Detoxification
Coffee substitute
Inflammation of the Liver

Recipes With Dandelion

FRITTERS

1/3 cup flour (can use GF)
1/3 cup almond flour
1 tsp tumeric powder
pinch of salt
1x egg
1/2 cup of milk
2 tbsp Coconut oil for cooking
Honey or maple syrup to serve

Mix flour, almond flour, salt, tumeric together, add whisked egg together in a bowl.

Mix well then add milk and mix into a batter.

Meanwhile heat the coconut oil in a saucepan.
Now to prepare your dandelions. One by one, cut the dandelion flower heads off their stems. Gradually place the flower heads into the batter to cover. Gently pick out and drop into the hot oil and cook for approx 5 minutes until browned. These taste delicious on their own or with a drizzle of honey.
Yummy goodness!!

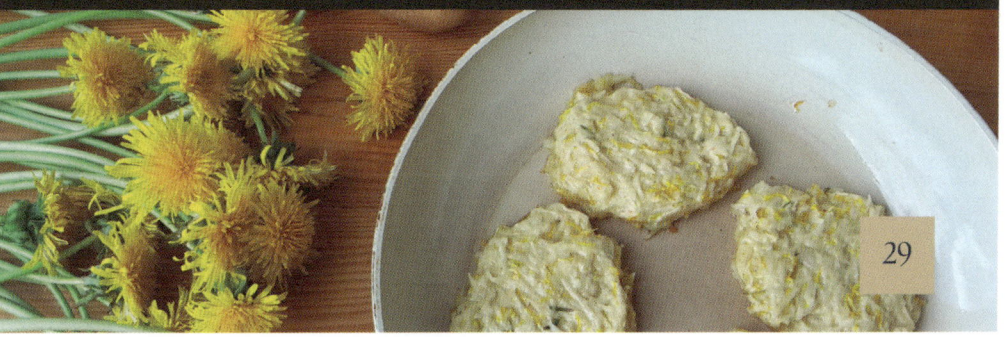

Recipes With Dandelion

SALAD
Add the leaves to a Spring greens salad with a dash of olive oil, lemon juice and garlic.

COOKED ROOTS
Saute a cup of dandelion roots cut into rings in 1 tblsp olive or coconut oil, add a little water and salt, cover and simmer. Serve with soya sauce.

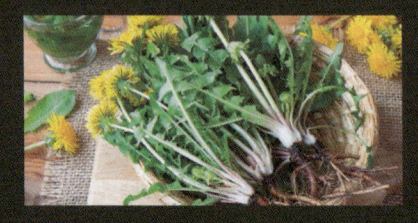

COFFEE
Wash and dry the roots thoroughly, preferably in the sunshine, then roast in the oven until they are brittle. Grind coarsely into powder and use as ordinary coffee. Alternatively just eat them neat when roasted.

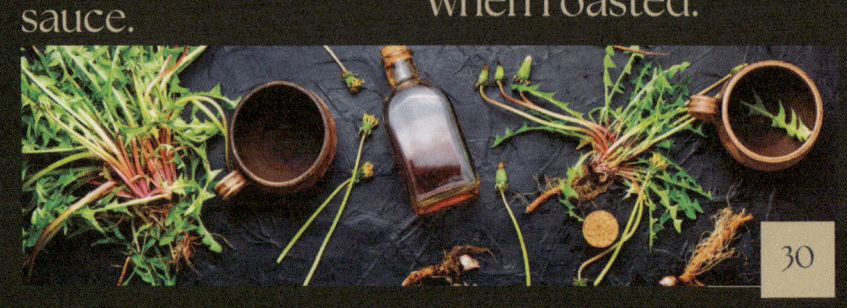

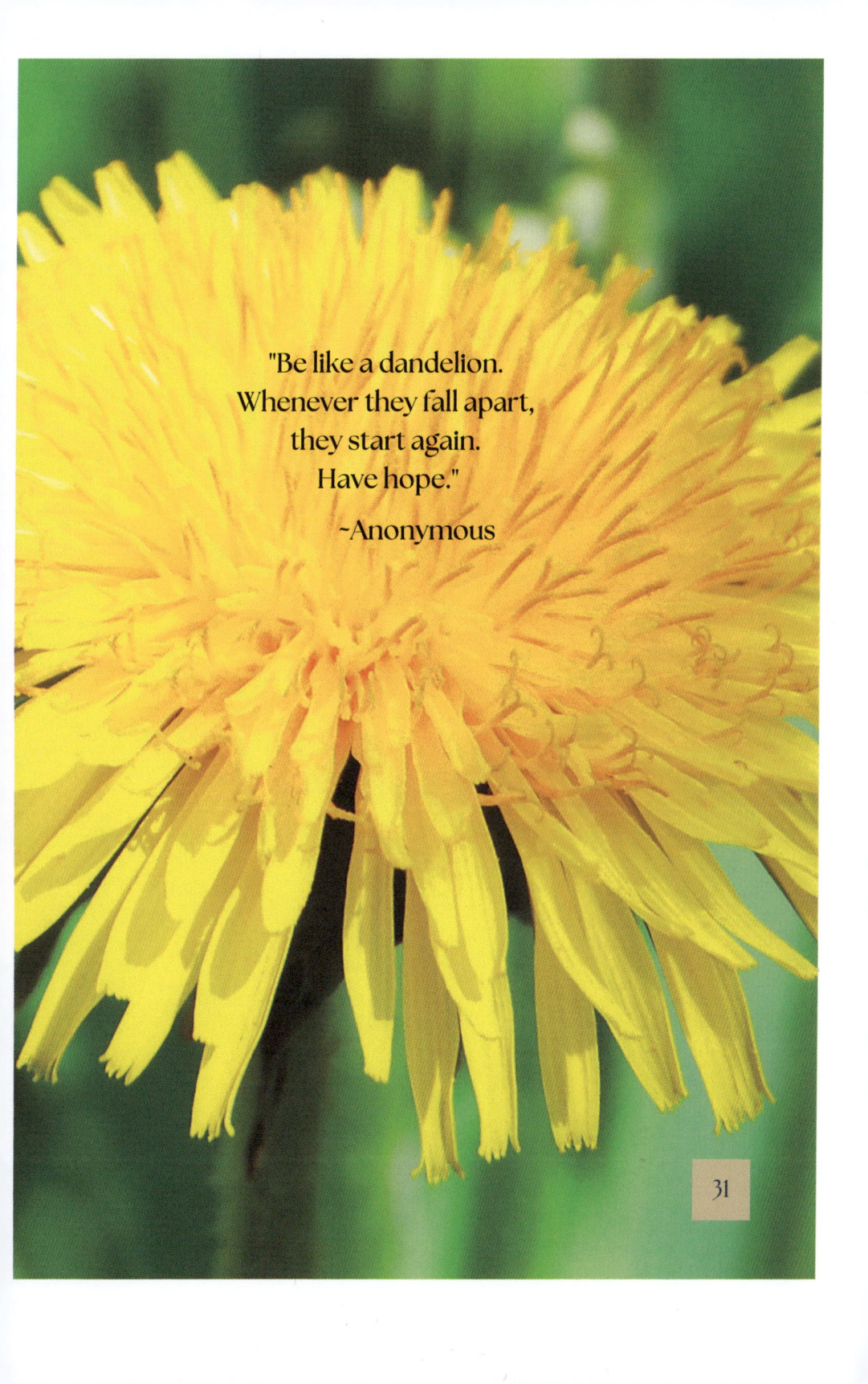

"Be like a dandelion.
Whenever they fall apart,
they start again.
Have hope."

~Anonymous

Some see a weed,
some see a wish.

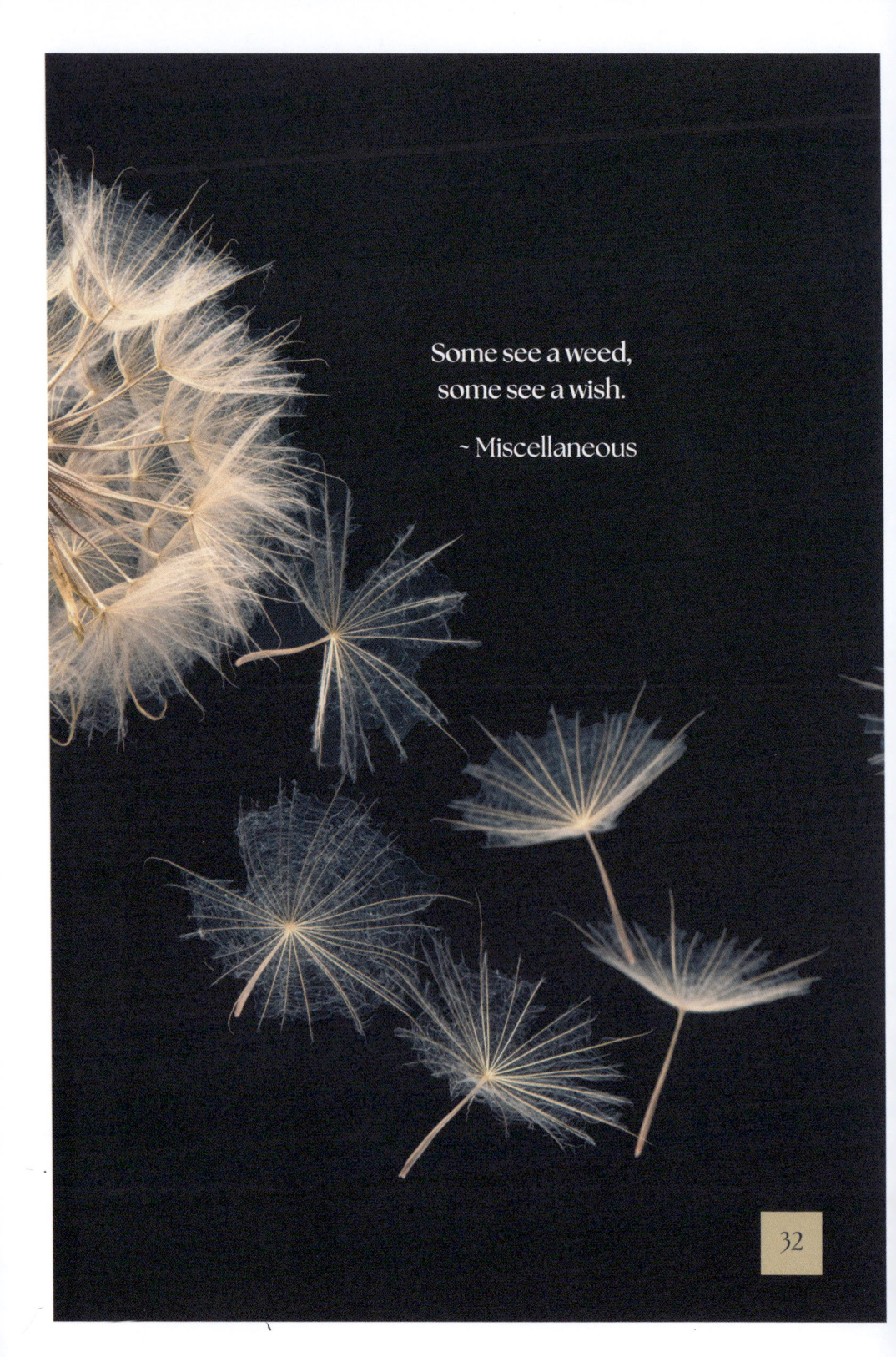

~ Miscellaneous

☾ CLEAVERS

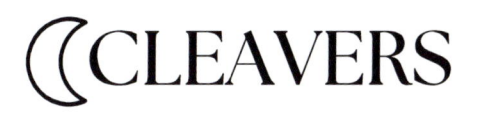

Latin Name: *Galium aparine*

Family Name: Rubiaceae family (Coffee, madder, bedstraw, gardinia, cinchona)

Other Names: Goosegrass, Clivers, sticky willy, scratch tongue, stick-a-back, and catchweed

Parts Used: all the plant

Habitat: field edges, woody, marshland

Identification: Fast growing creeper with narrow pointed leaves that grow in whorls of 6-8 around square stems. The plant is covered in tiny prickles. Grows 50-150cm high.

History & Folklore

Considered a potent love medicine by some Native American tribes and believed to be auspicious for a woman to bathe in cleavers to attract love into her life. An amazing detoxifier, even Plato referred to this plant for its usefulness in promoting weightloss.

High in vitamin C, this is a much loved weed by children, used in traditional games 'tag' games. As a hair rinse it makes the hair grow long and strong. In the middle ages it was used for poisonous spider bites.

Traditionally used with milk, even today in Sweden, fresh milk is strained through a straw bed of fresh cleavers which is believed to clean it of impurities and imbue the milk with its healing properties.

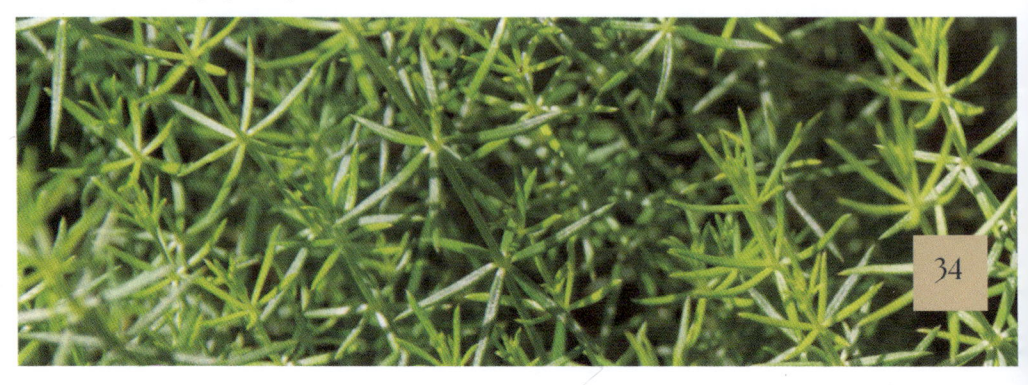

Healing Properties

Depurative

Diuretic

Astringent

Febrifuge

Blood cleanser

Tonic

Alterative

Aperient

Anti-inflammatory

Anti-cancer

Detoxification

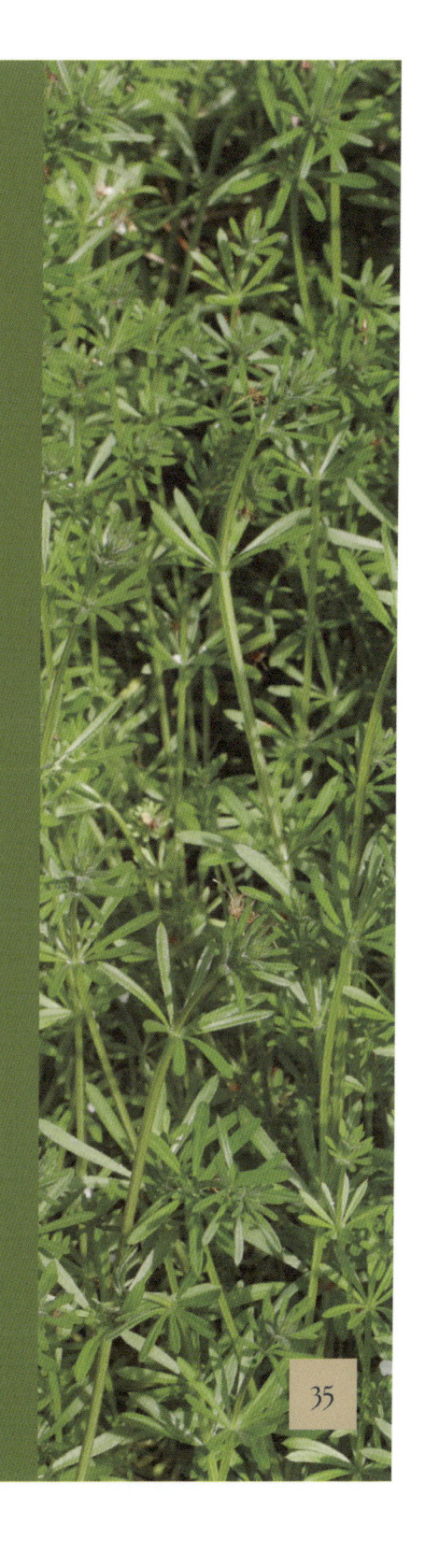

Medicinal Uses

Oedema

Swellings

Obesity

Swollen Glands

Urinary tract infections

Reduces fevers

Psoriasis

Eczema

Cystitis

Dandruff

Tumours

Lymphatic drainage

Warning: can cause dermatitis in some individuals when applied externally. Avoid if diabetic.

Recipes With Cleavers

JUICE

Fresh young cleavers shoots collected in Spring before they become too hard and stringy can be added by the handful to any juice and are easily put through a juicer. Aids lymphatic drainage as part of a Spring detox in any juice.

DETOXIFICATION

Drink as a juice everyday for 5 weeks, to encourage weight loss.

VEGETABLE

Briefly boiled or steamed as a green vegetable, makes a healthy addition to any meal. Also incredibly tasty in omelettes. The tender shoots are delicious added to salads.

POULTICE

Pound the fresh herb in a pestle and mortar and apply directly to skin swellings, tumours and even ulcers.

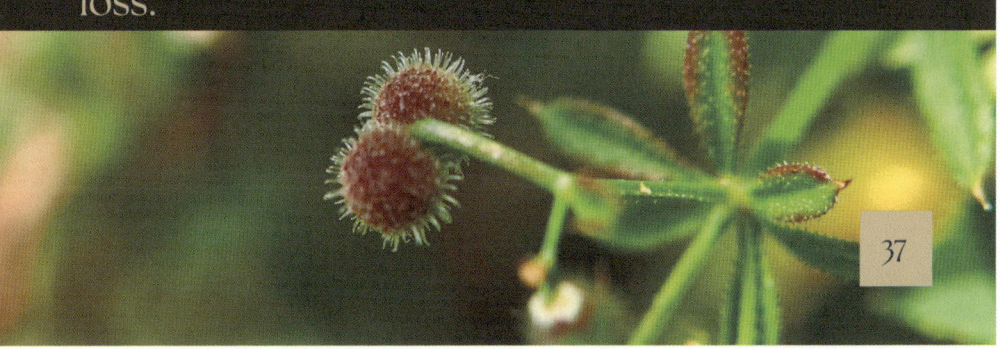

Recipes With Cleavers

COFFEE
Collect the little round ball shaped seeds and gently roast in the oven on the lowest oven temperature for 10-20 minutes. Grind up or pound in a pestle and mortar and use as a non-caffeinated coffee substitute. Cleavers is related to coffee, being a member of the same family, rubiaceae.

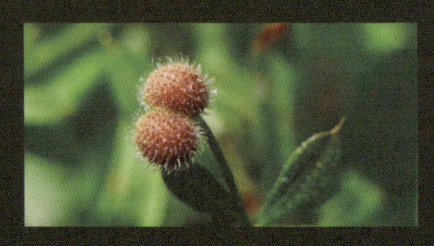

TEA
Dry the collected fresh shoots. Cut them up and pop a small handful into a teapot, add off-the-boil water, leave to seep for 5 minutes and drink this totally cleansing tea. Very useful for urinary tract infections.

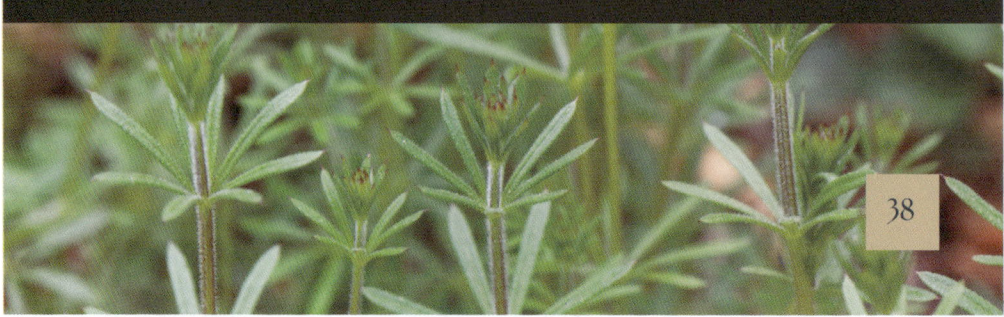

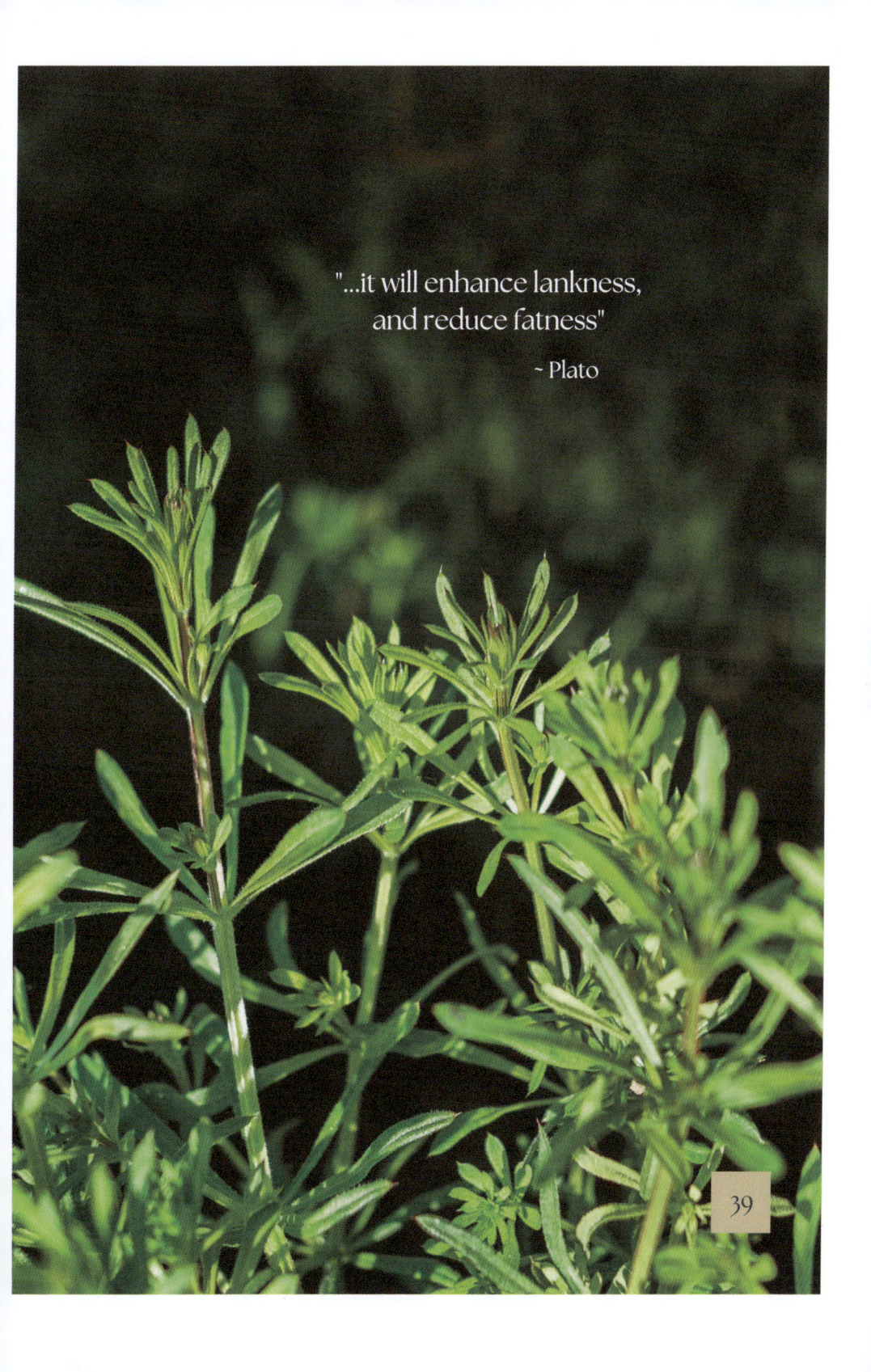

> "...it will enhance lankness,
> and reduce fatness"
>
> ~ Plato

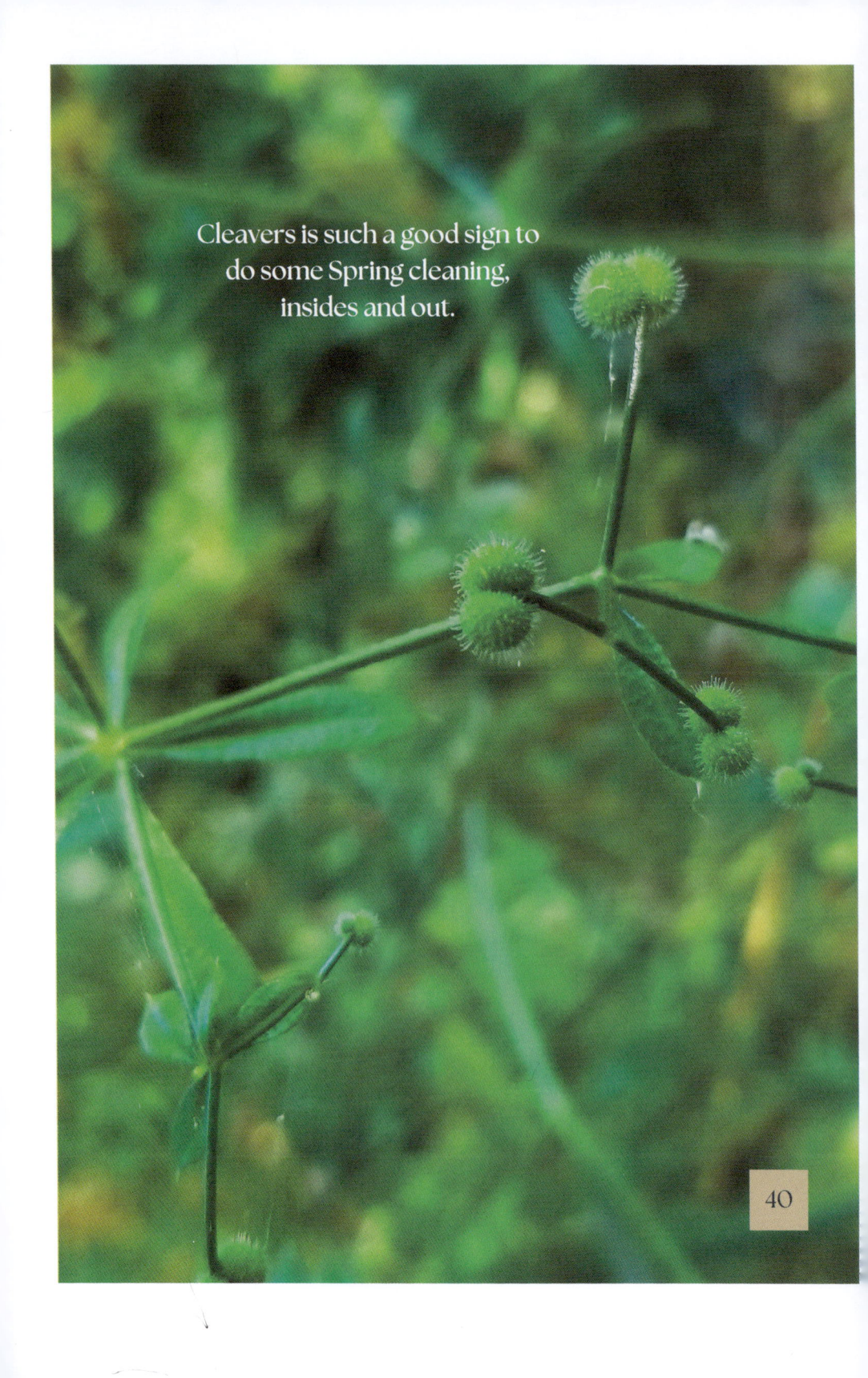

Cleavers is such a good sign to do some Spring cleaning, insides and out.

☾ CHICKWEED

Latin Name: *Stellaria media*

Family Name: Caryophyllaceae family (Campions, bladder campion, soapwort, sweet williams)

Other Names: common chickweed

Parts Used: all of the plant

Habitat: field edges, anywhere in the world, available all year round

Identification: Chickweed tends to creep. It has stiff, hairy, mouse eared leaves with beautiful star shaped white flowers. There are many varieties such as woodruff and bedstraw.

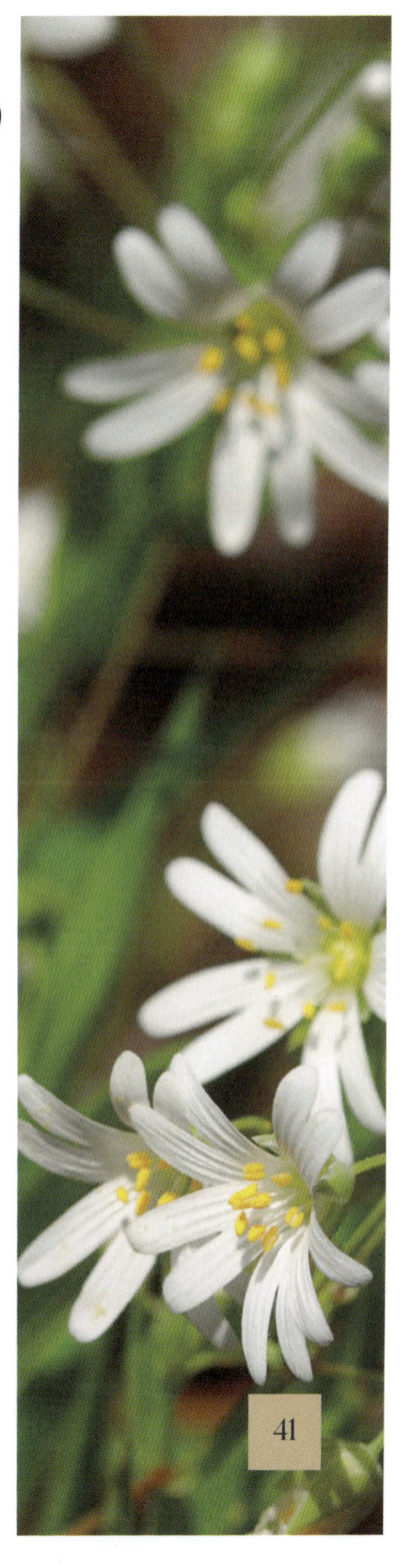

Folklore & History

As the name suggests chickweed is loved by chickens. There is not a place on the planet that has not been blessed with chickweed for the seeds travel.

The latin name 'stellaria media' means medium sized star. In an emergency this truely is a star remedy. Chickweed is considered a magical plant, associated with relationships, fidelity and love. A sprig of chickweed in your pocket attracts love and popping some in your partners dish ensured a strong relationship.

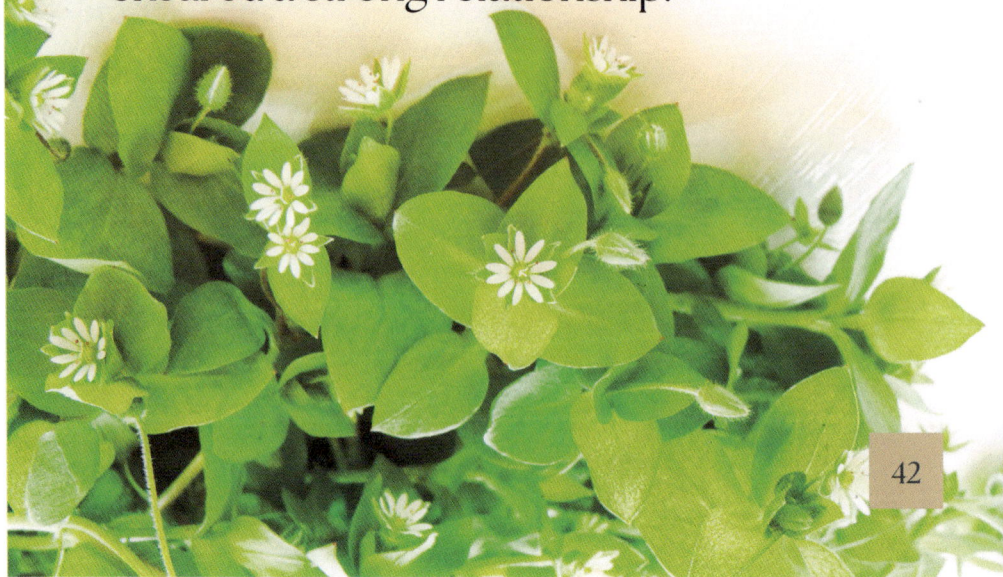

Therapeutic Use

Vulnerary

Anti-rheumatic

Demulcent

Refrigerant

Emollient

Antipruritic

Antioxidant

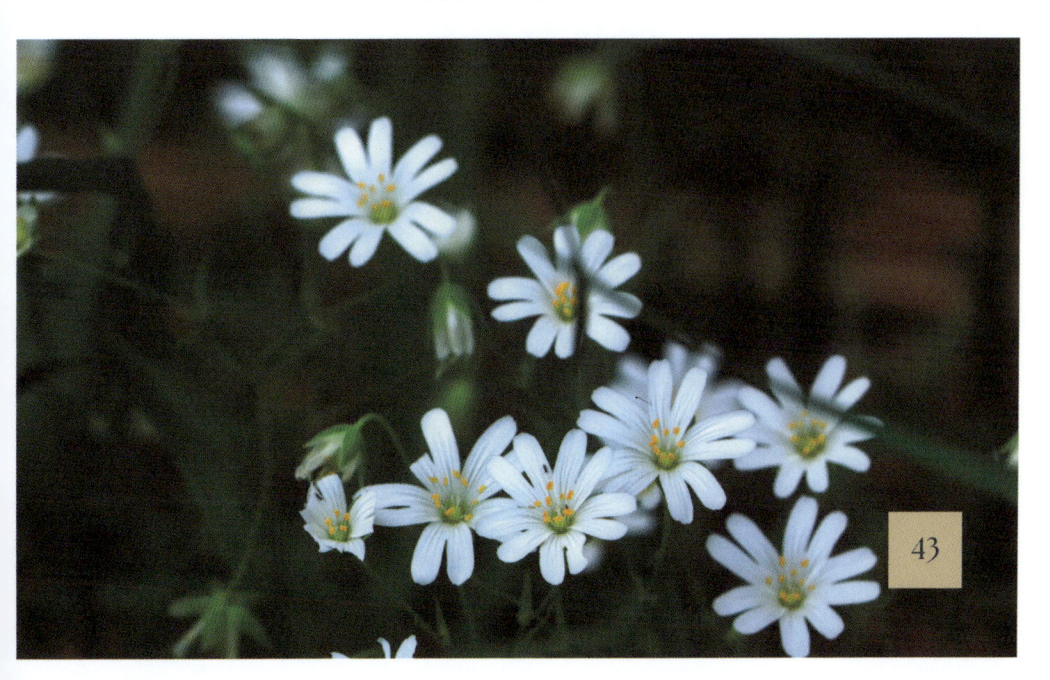

Medicinal Uses

Ulcers and Abscesses
Coughing
Burns
Chillblains
Inflamed skin
Skin Rashes
Itchiness
Constipation
Wasp & Bee stings
Scratches & scrapes
Poison ivy burns
Eczema & Psoriasis

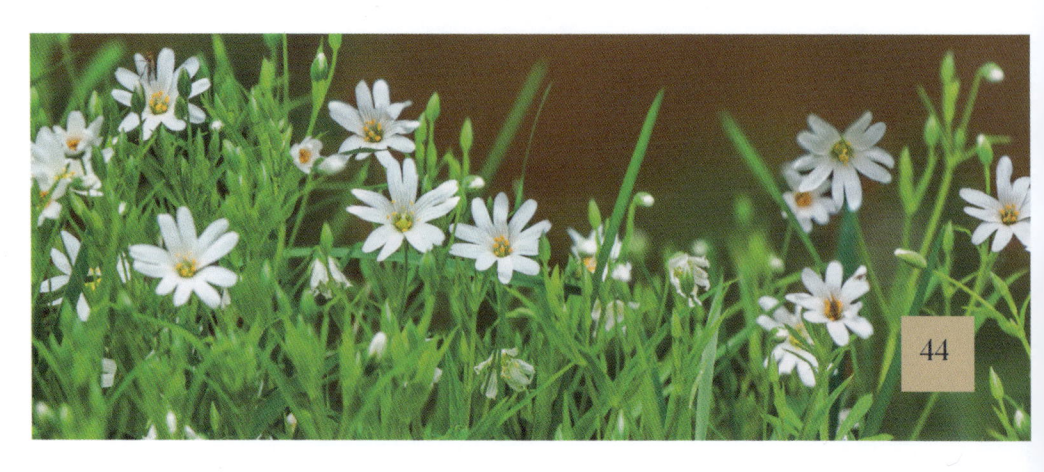

Recipes With Chickweed

EGG & CHICKWEED SANDWICH

Handful of freshly picked chickweed
1x egg
A splash of vinegar
Mayonnaise optional
Slices of bread
Seasoning

Wash and dry the chickweed. Put the egg in a saucepan of water with a dash of vinegar and leave to boil.
Boil it for 5 minutes to hard boil the egg. Remove the egg carefully with a spoon. When cooled, crack it open and completely remove the shell.

With a fork mash up the egg in a bowl, then add a tablespoon of mayonnaise if desired, a teaspoon of mustard works too if you like it spicy.

Cut up the fresh chickweed, season and lather on two slices of bread and make your sandwich.

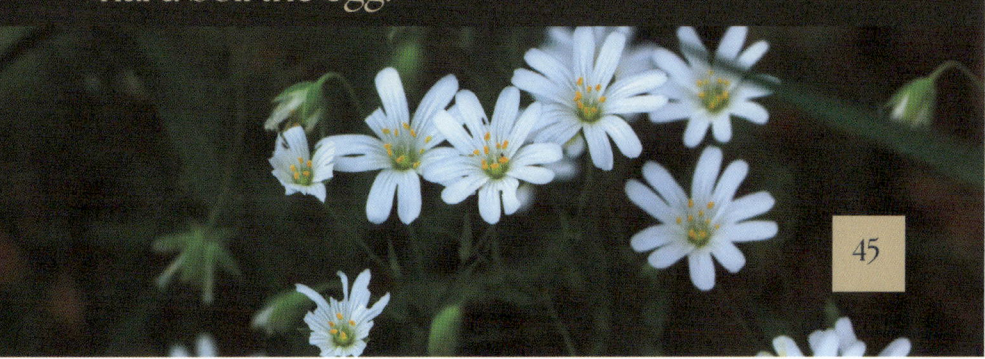

Recipes With Chickweed

POLTICE
Either pound these in a pestle and mortar or food processor. However when in emergencies, when out in the field, simply grab and chew them up with your teeth and apply directly to wounds, fresh cuts, grazes, scraps insect stings and bites.
Fantastic First Aid!

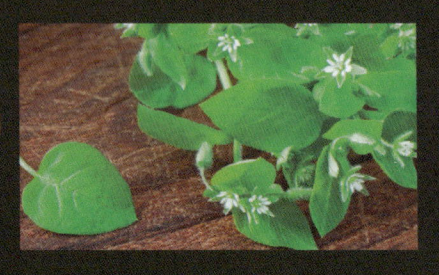

SPRING SALAD
Such a tasty Spring green, lovely addition to salads, refreshing, and delicious.

FOR THE GARDEN
Chickweed grows in PH neutral soil so a great indicator for keen gardeners.

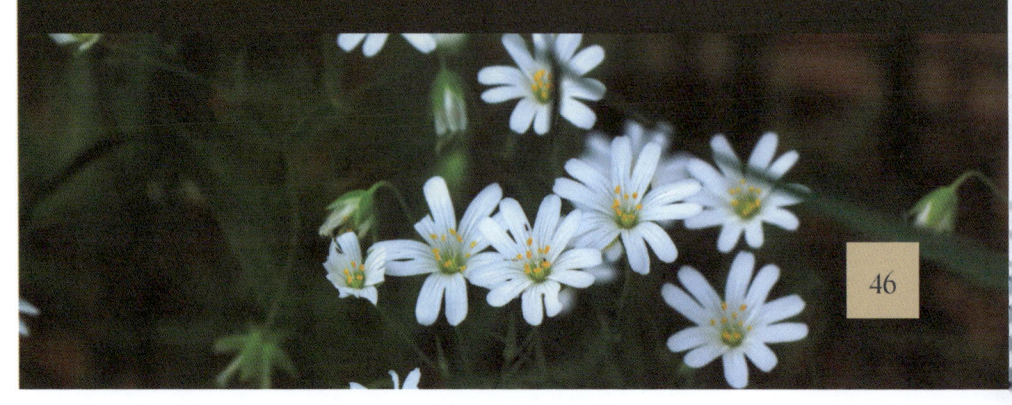

"....rubbing it well with your hand, and bind also some of the herb, if you choose, to the place, and with God's blessing it will help in three times dressing."

~ Culpepper

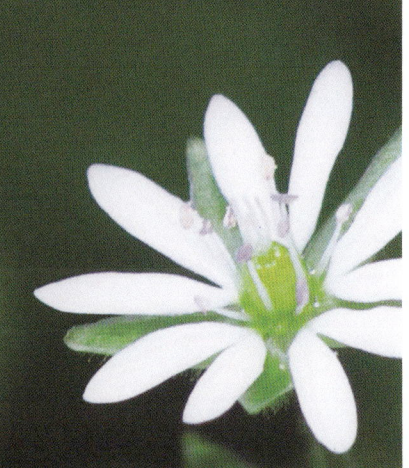

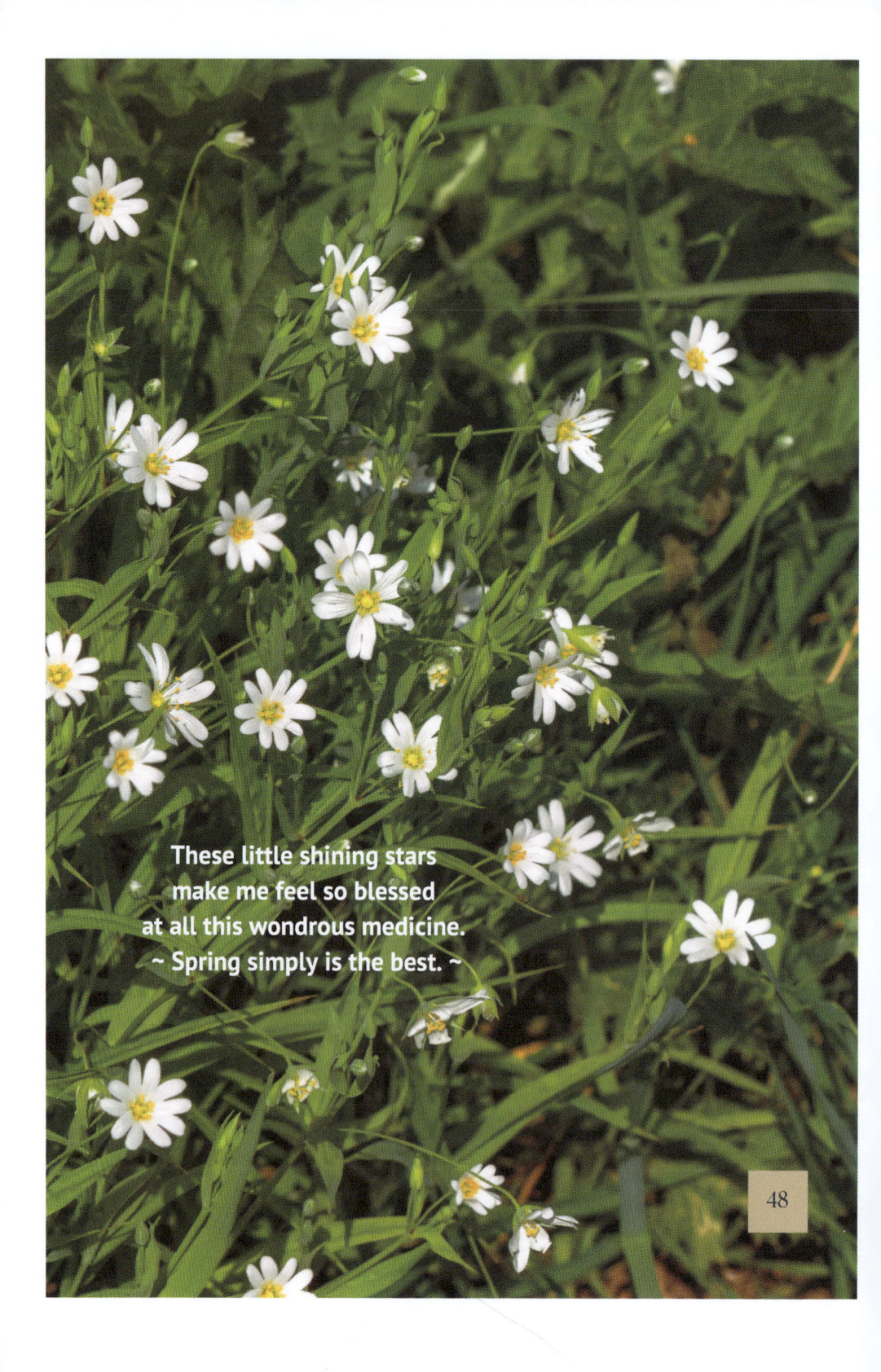

These little shining stars
make me feel so blessed
at all this wondrous medicine.
~ Spring simply is the best. ~

♀ VIOLET

Latin Name: *Viola odorata*

Family Name: Violaceae family (Heartsease, pansies, violets)

Other Names: Sweet violet, violette de mars, march violet

Parts Used: flowers and leaves

Habitat: shade, walls, hedge banks, lawns

Identification: Downy heart shaped leaves with long stalks. Flowers purple, lilac, white, blue with hooked stigma. Self fertilising, it flowers in Spring and again in Autumn.

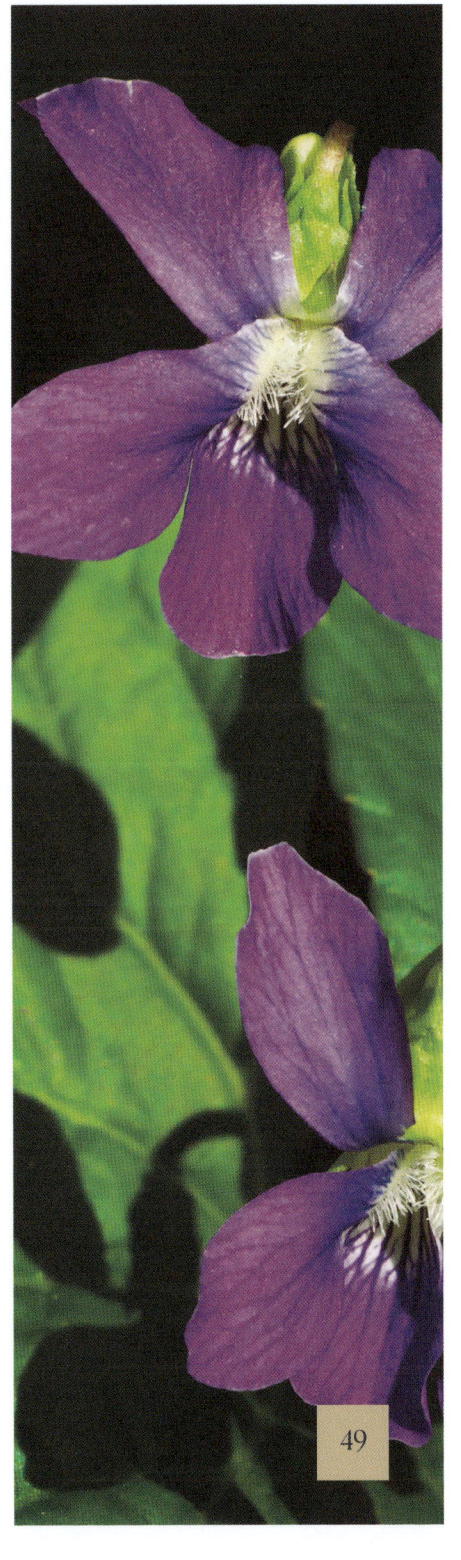

Folklore & History

A myth about violet involve a beautiful nymph called Io who caught the eye of the king of Gods. Zeus and her had an affair whilst he was married to Hera. In order for Hera to not find out as she was a very jealous wife, Zeus turned Io into a heifer/young cow for her camouflage.

So Io as a heifer on eating grass finds that the grass was much too harsh for her so she just cried and cried and cried.

She was so upset about being a heifer and then eating the grass that was much too harsh for her to ingest.

So Zeus turned her tears into violets. So everywhere she went she cried violets that she was then able to eat.

Folklore & History

Hera found out about Io and in her jealousy sent a fly to 'bug' this heifer. Io then travelled the world crying her tears wherever she went.

When finally she got to Egypt, she managed to release the spell, turned back into a human and married a king. Later on she became known as Isis and worshipped as the Goddess Isis.

The violet is a symbol of humility, love, faithfulness and modesty. Carrying a violet in your pocket will bring you luck and protection.

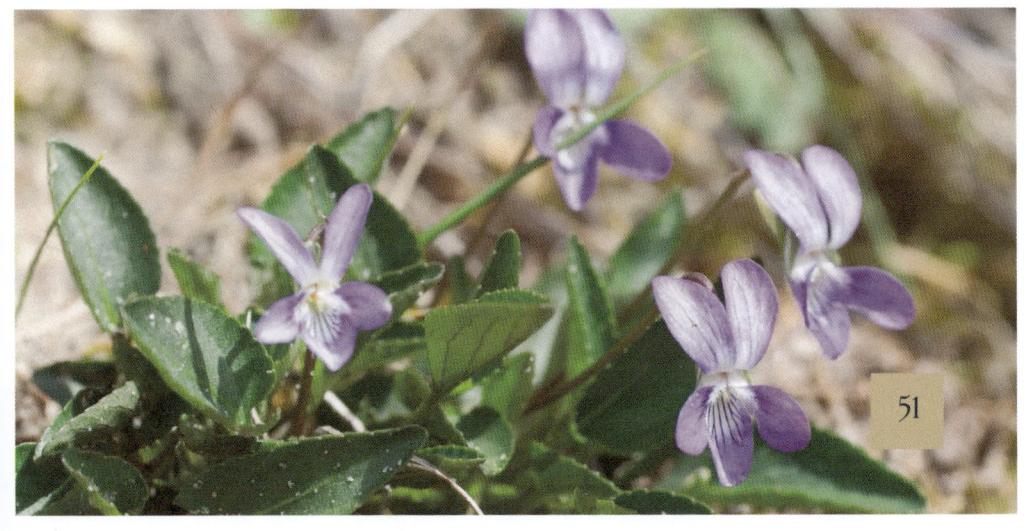

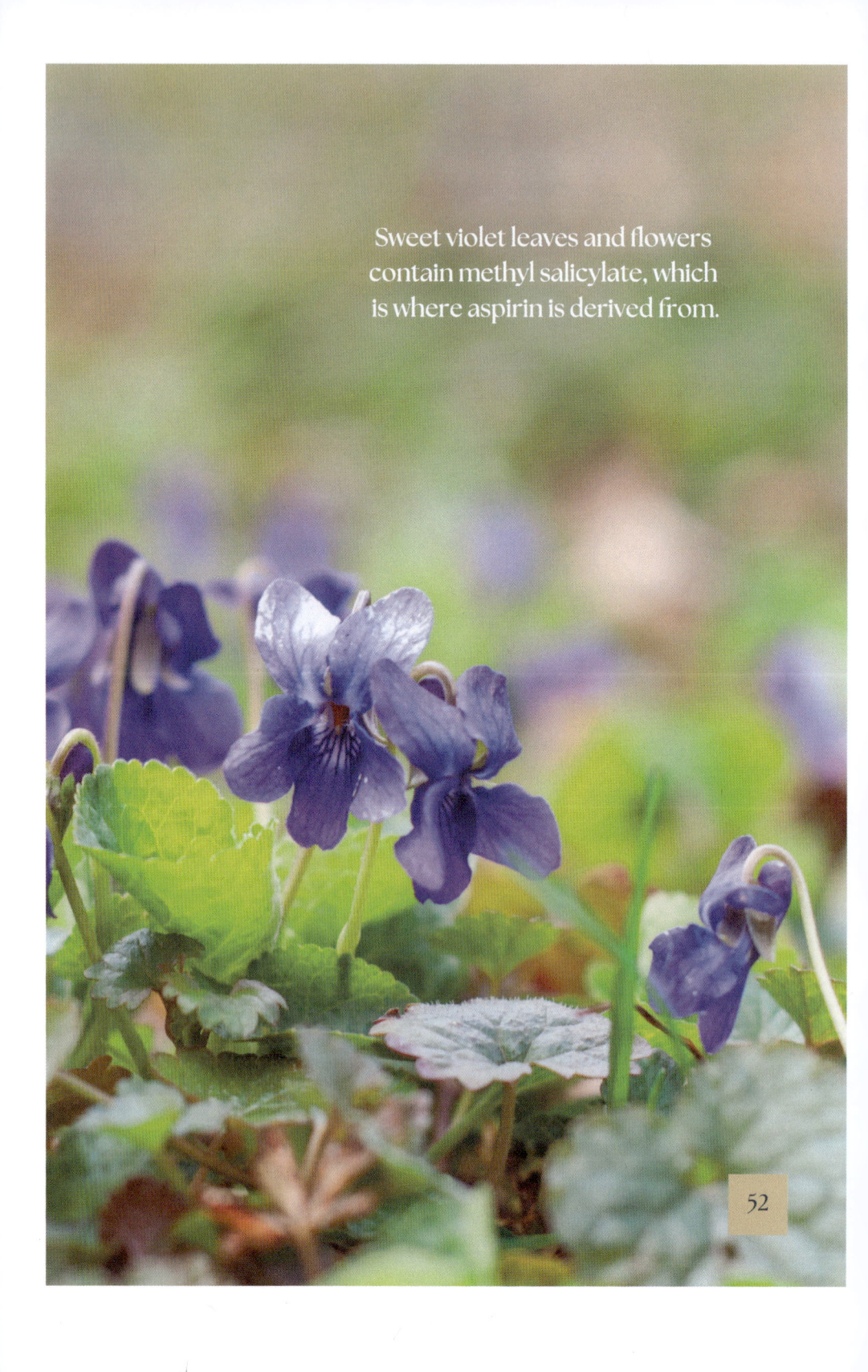

Sweet violet leaves and flowers contain methyl salicylate, which is where aspirin is derived from.

Therapeutic Uses

Antiseptic

Expectorant

Anti-inflammatory

Diuretic

Antimicrobial

Analgesic

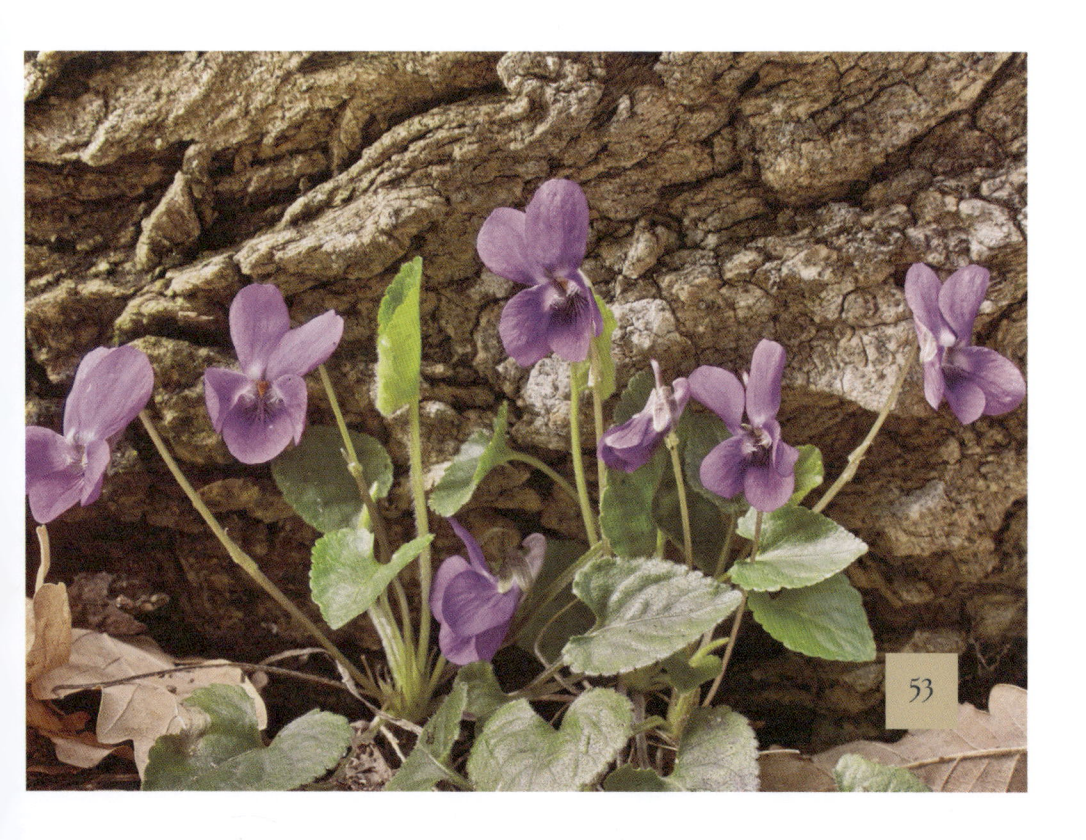

Medicinal Uses

Hangovers

Coughs

Colds

Catarrh

Bronchial

Mild laxative complaints

Migraines

Headaches

Skin inflammation

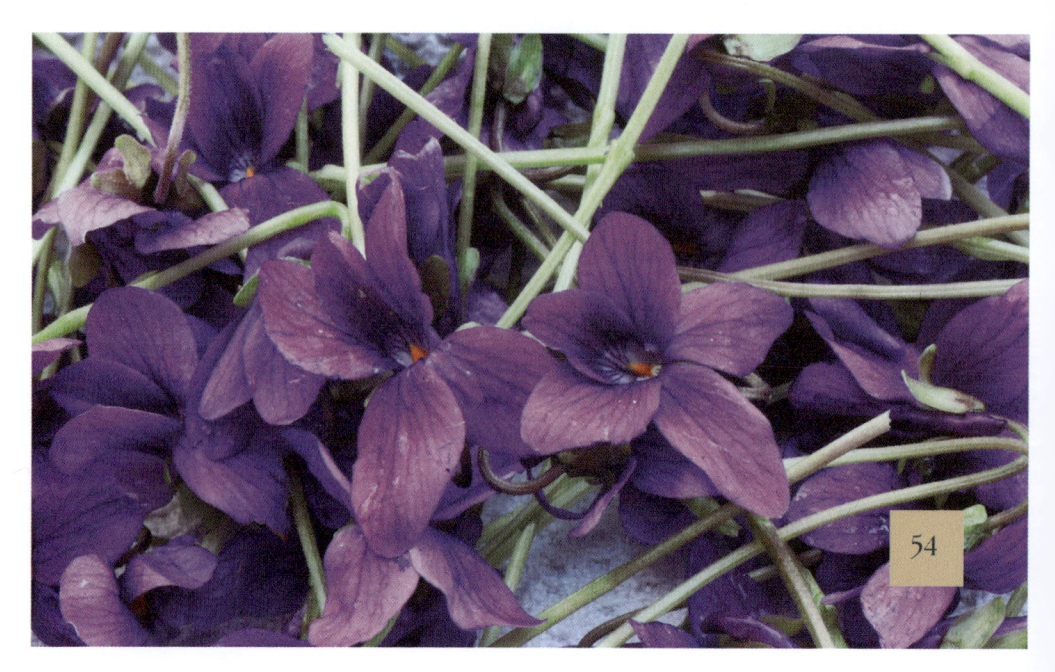

Recipes With Violets

SYRUP

2-3 cups of fresh flowers
1/2 pint boiling water approx
500gm sugar (we use coconut)

Remove all the leaves and green bits and pop the flowers in a bain marie, cover with boiling water and leave overnight to steep.

The next day, add sugar to the violets in water. Heat water underneath bain marie to a rolling boil, stirring until all the sugar dissolves. Once this happens, remove from the heat, cool, strain and bottle. This is a great remedy for chesty coughs and colds and as a mild laxative for small children.

I have also made this syrup with honey (1x cupful). Note, this syrup should be a beautiful lilac, purpley blue colour.

Use the syrup on ice cream, in cookies/biscuits, cakes or just take it by the spoon, whatever you prefer.

If you don't have a bain marie, a simple set up of a small saucepan half full with water with a pyrex glass dish on top works perfectly well.

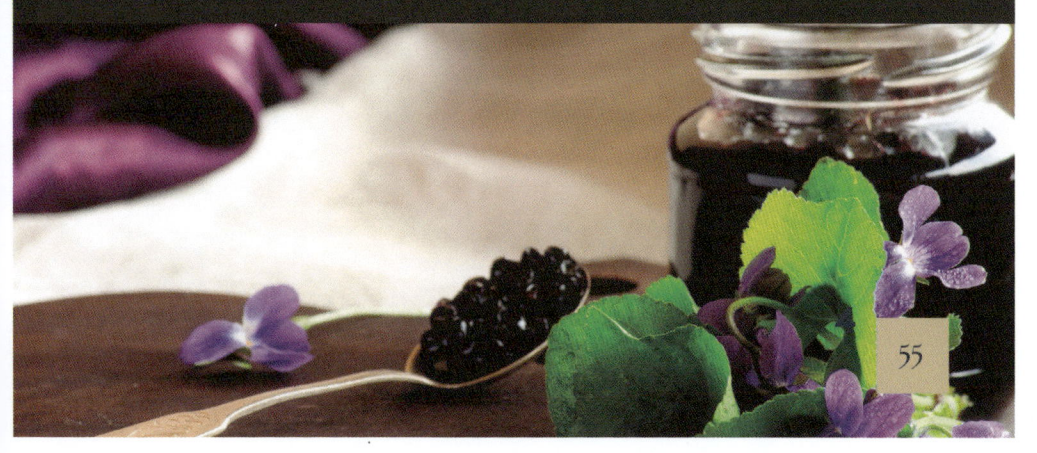

Recipes With Violets

VIOLET PUDDING (Vyolette)

2 cups of violet petals washed
1 cup of water
1+1/2 cup milk (I used almond)
2-3 tblsp flour (I used rice/almond)
4 tsp sugar (coconut sugar)
1/4 tsp saffron (optional)

In a saucepan, bring water to a boil. Stir in violet petals, return to the boil. Stir constantly for 1 minute. Use a sieve, drain, press out all water and keep separately. Then mash the cooked petals to a paste.

In a saucepan bring milk to a boil, reduce heat, and simmer, stir for 2 minutes. Add mashed petals. Stir in flour, a bit at a time, then sugar and saffron. Continue to simmer and stir for 5 minutes. Serve in individual small bowls.

Tastes like oatmeal. This is a 14th Century recipe. Drink water as a tisane.

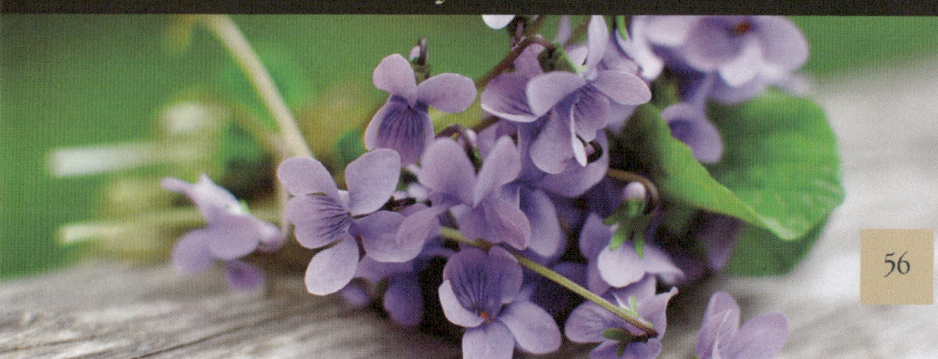

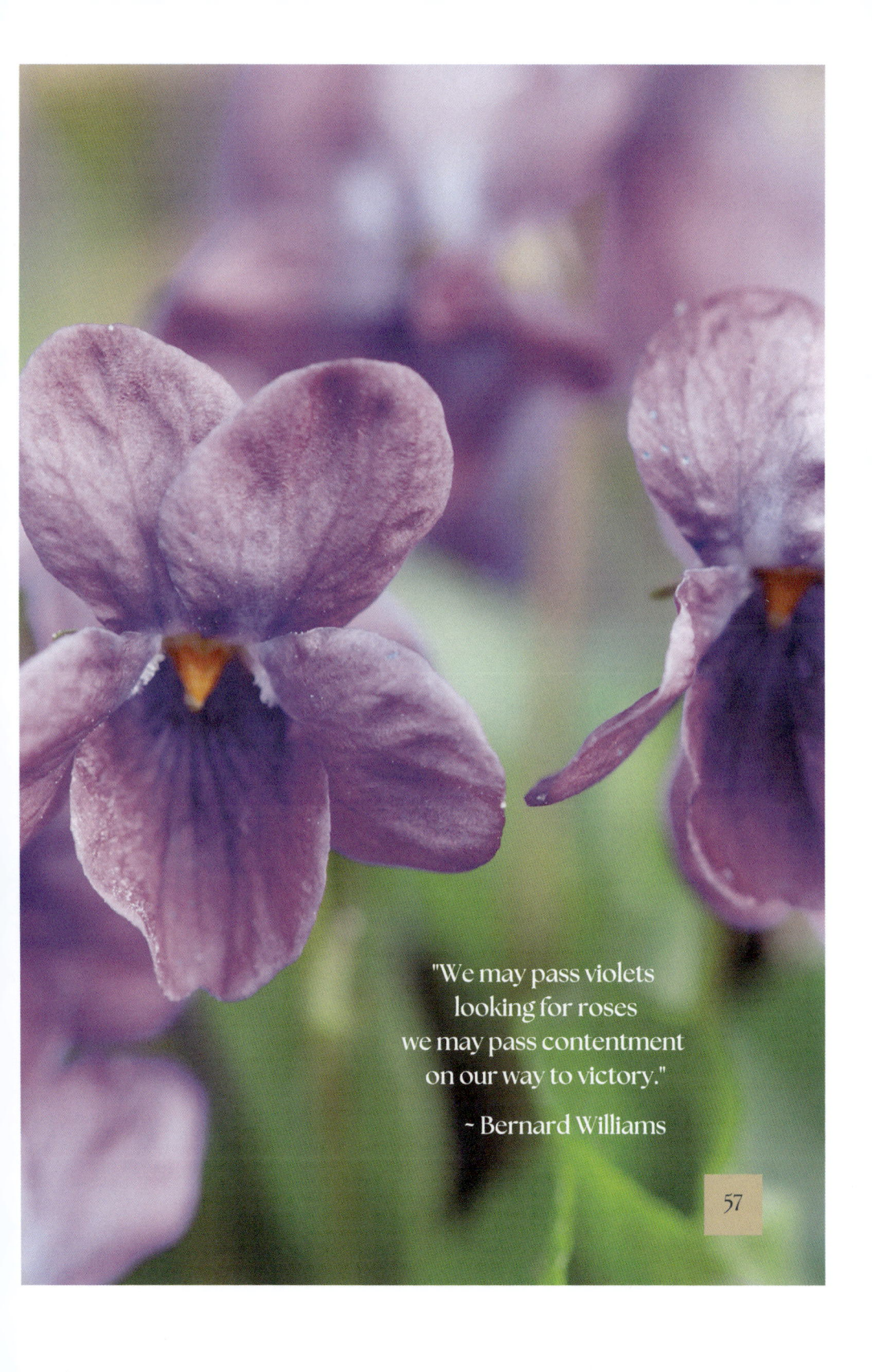

"We may pass violets
looking for roses
we may pass contentment
on our way to victory."

~ Bernard Williams

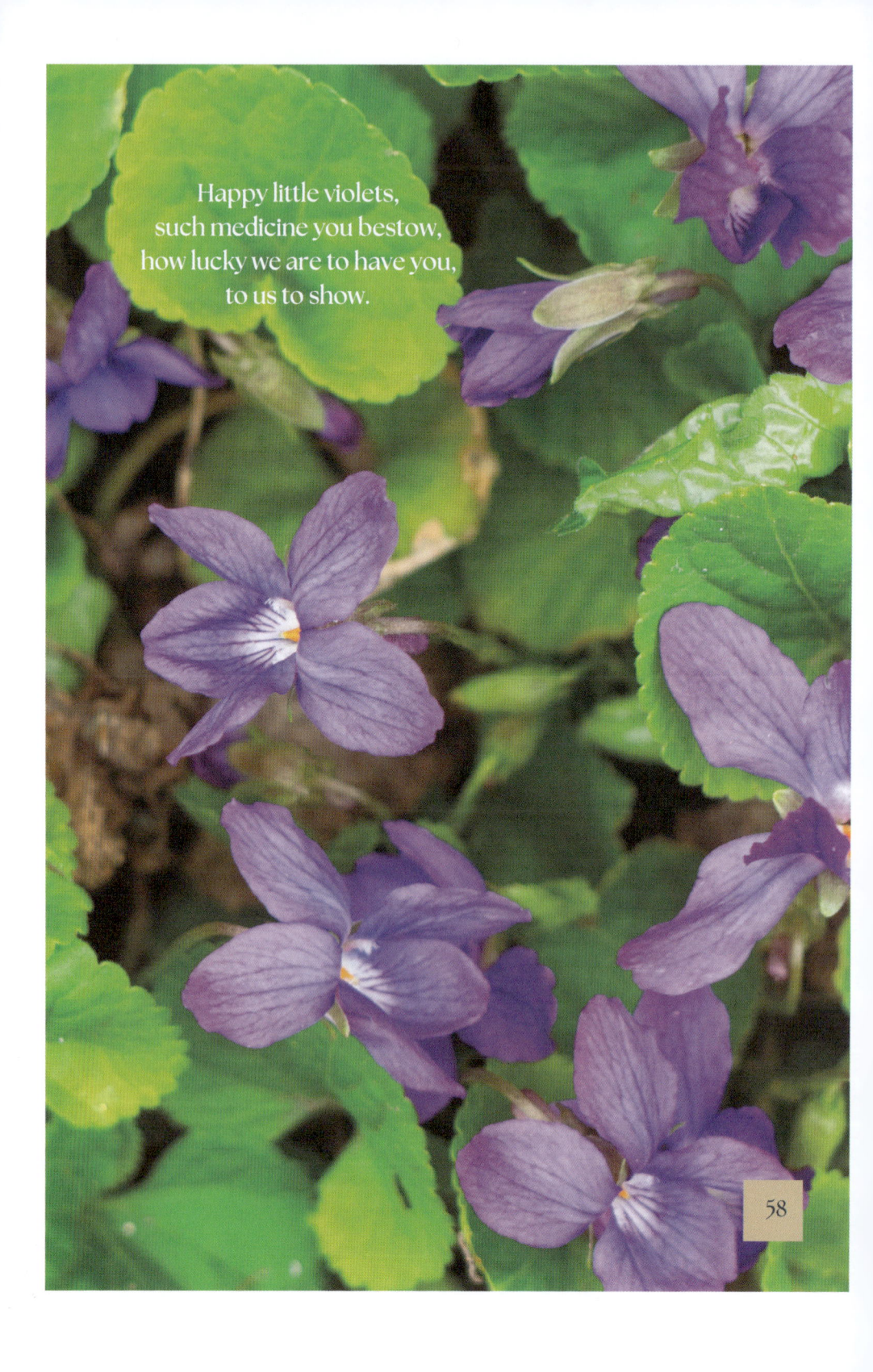

Happy little violets,
such medicine you bestow,
how lucky we are to have you,
to us to show.

♂ PLANTAIN

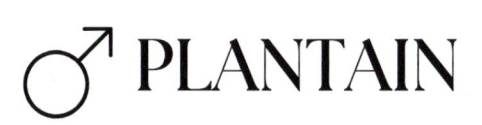

Latin Name: Plantago spp major and lanceolata

Family Name: Plantaginaceae family
(Speedwell, purslane, foxglove)

Other Names: Rats tail, Ribwort

Parts Used: leaves, seeds

Habitat: field edges, woods, marshland

Identification: Oval leaves are strongly veined in a basal rosette narrowing into a long tap root. Tiny yellowish-green flowers with purple and yellow anthers in a spike.

Same family as the digestive aid psyllium, another most useful species.

History & Folklore

Plantago has a long history, having survived 3 ice ages. Native American Indians call it 'white mans foot' for they grew wherever the white man walked and worked. Interestingly, the name comes from the latin 'planta' meaning 'sole of the foot'.

The physicians of Myddfai, traditional welsh herbalists recommended compresses for respiratory complaints.

In mythology, plantain was a girl on the side of the road waiting for her lover, she waited so long, she turned into plantain. Christianity took it as a symbol of the path towards Christ.

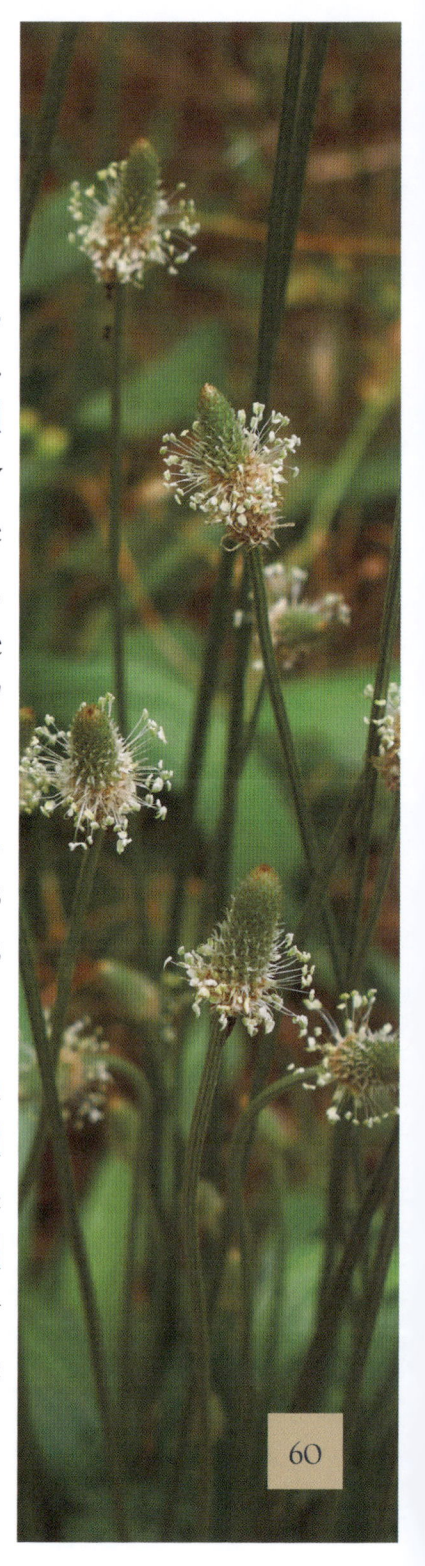

Therapeutic Uses

Anti-inflammatory

Muscilaginous

Analgesic

Antiseptic

Antihistamine

Antispasmodic

Diuretic

Antioxidant

Immunomodulating

Anti-Haemorragic

Hypoglycaemic

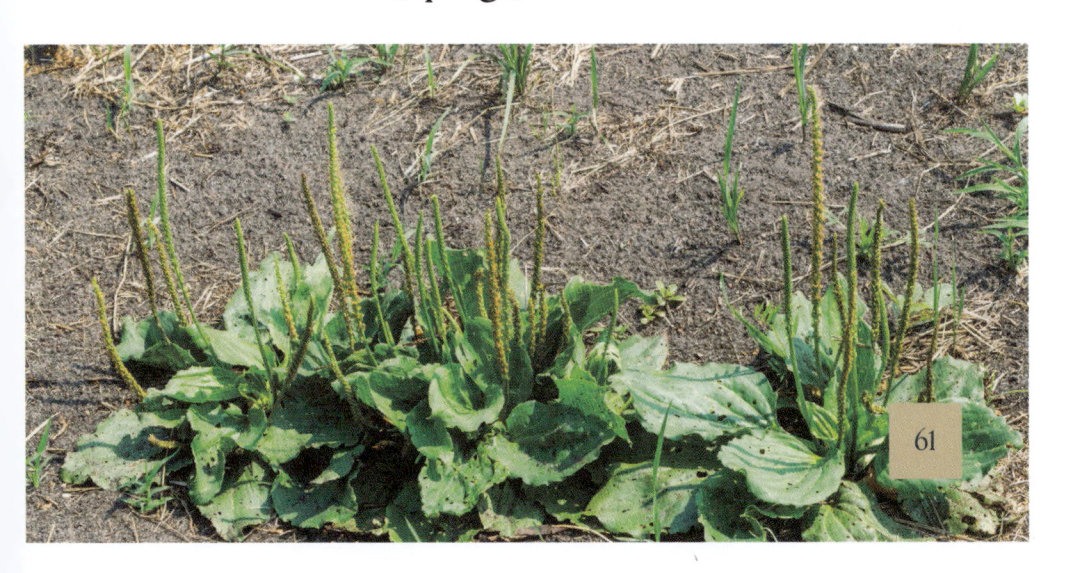

Medicinal Uses

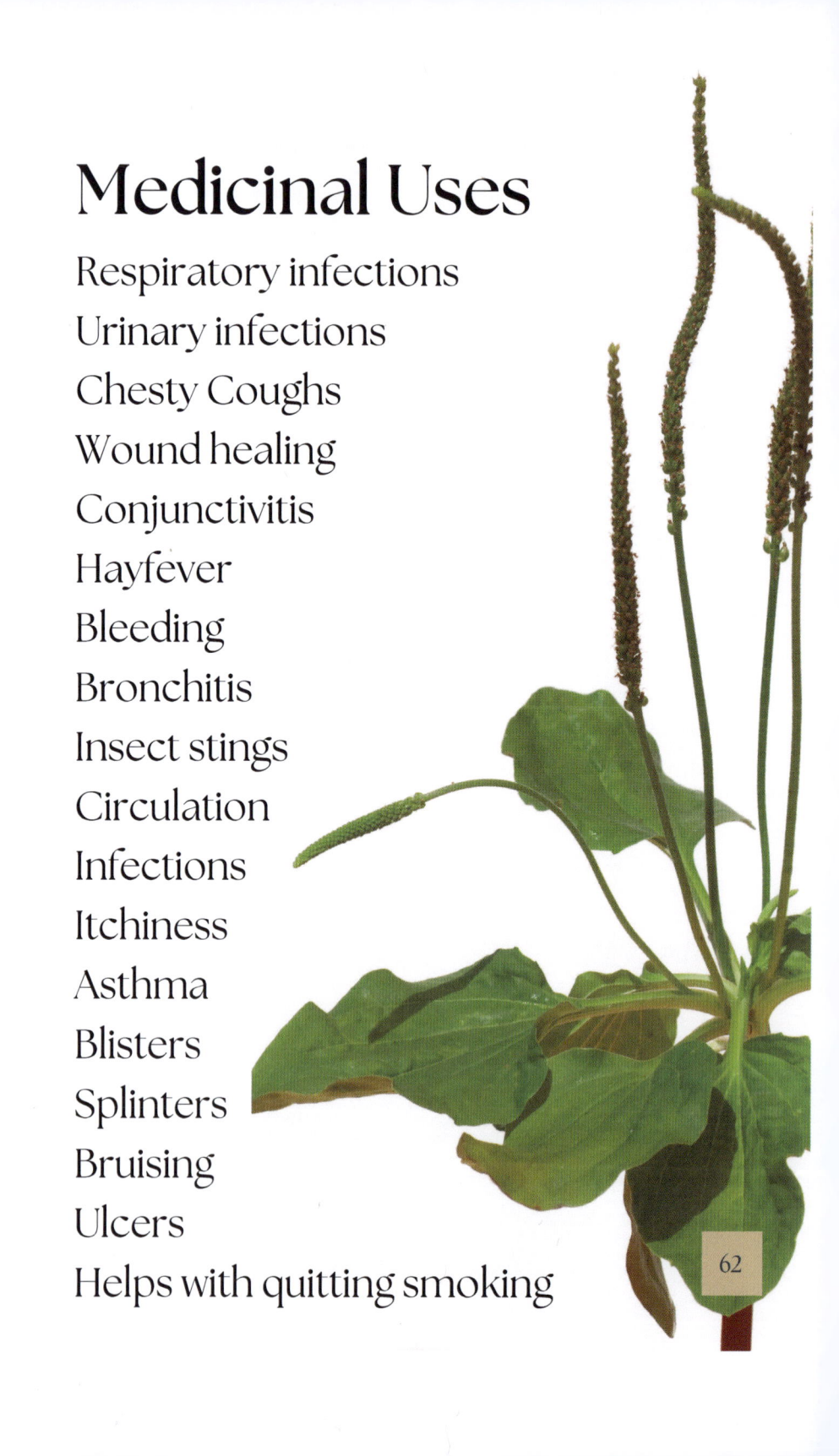

Respiratory infections
Urinary infections
Chesty Coughs
Wound healing
Conjunctivitis
Hayfever
Bleeding
Bronchitis
Insect stings
Circulation
Infections
Itchiness
Asthma
Blisters
Splinters
Bruising
Ulcers
Helps with quitting smoking

Recipes With Plantain

COOKING WITH PLANTAIN

I will not lie to you when i say it is a herb for survival and not one of choice in regards to it's palatability. That is until you smell it after cooking. Wow! it smells of truffle oil so it can happily flavour any dish with the exquisite aroma. It is highly nutritious containing calcium, vitamins A, C, and K. Cook as you would spinach.

MOISTURISER

Crush fresh plantain leaves in a pestle and mortar or in your hands. Cover your hands in the juice, they will feel remarkably soft. Can also be applied as a face mask.

INFUSED OIL

Cut up fresh plantain leaves and place them in a jar, fill the jar up with olive oil to cover the herb. Leave to sit in direct sunlight for a minimum 2-4 weeks. Strain before use.

Recipes With Plantain

FIRST AID

By far one of the most useful herbs when you are in need of some emergency first aid from your plant allies.

For bee, wasp stings or mosquito and spider bites, crush the leaves and apply the juice to the area and wrap leaves around as a bandage.

For any scraps, cuts and bleeding, crush the leaves and apply the juice and crushed herb to the affected area.

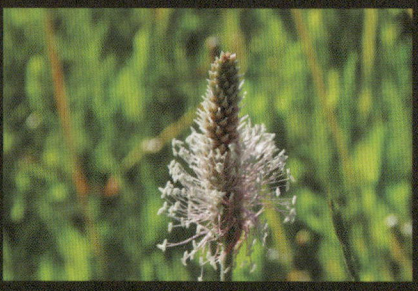

In emergencies this is the first plant I look for. to rip up the leaves and chew them. They are hugely antiseptic.

FEET

Place under the feet to relax and restore tired and aching feet.

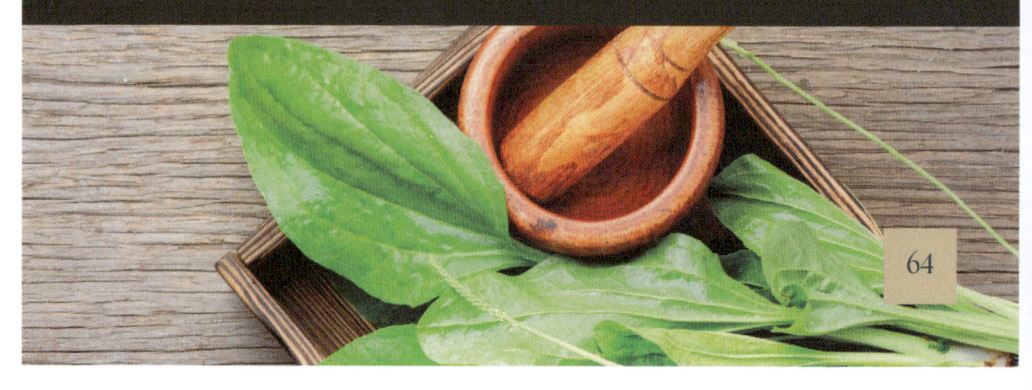

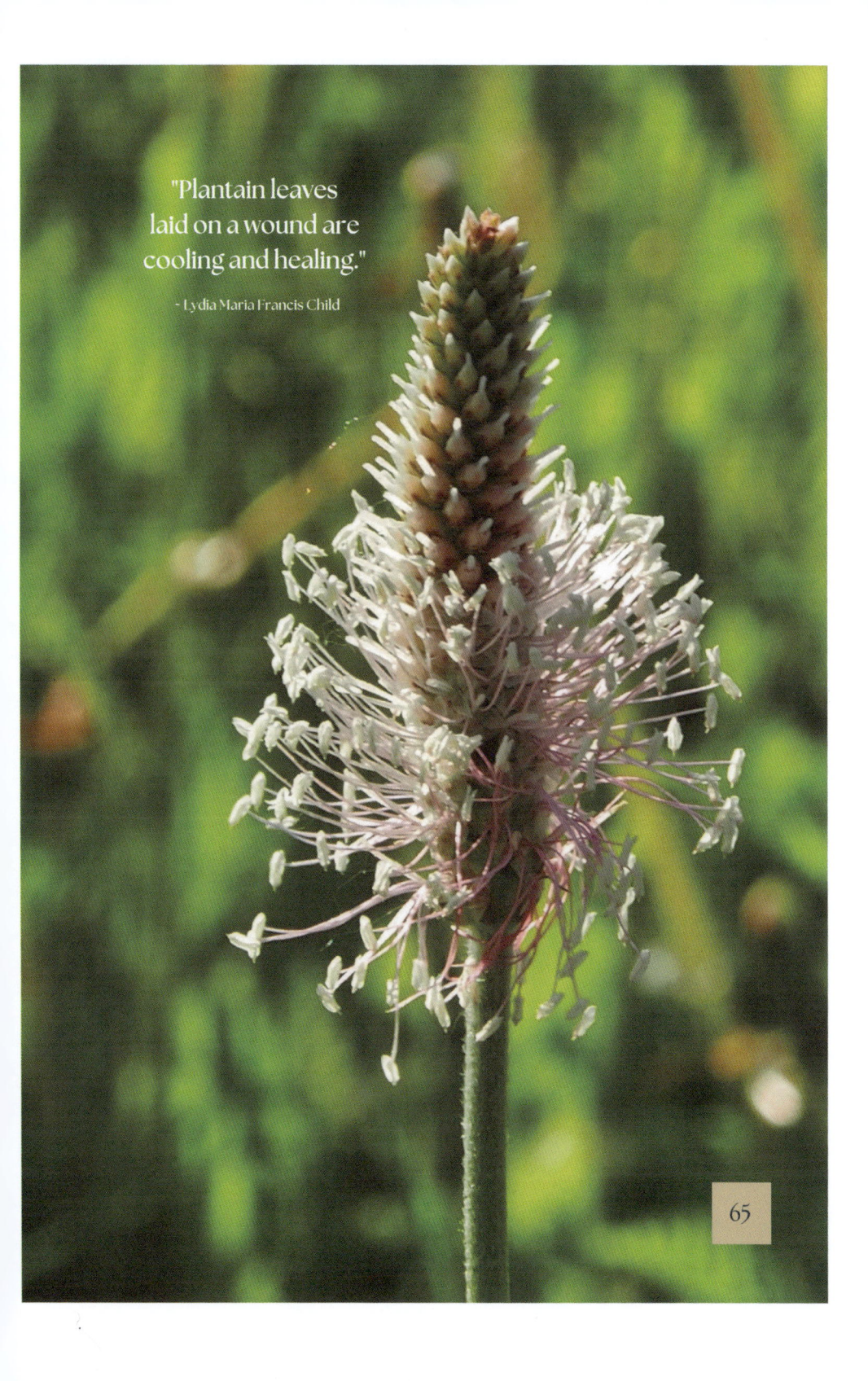

"Plantain leaves
laid on a wound are
cooling and healing."

- Lydia Maria Francis Child

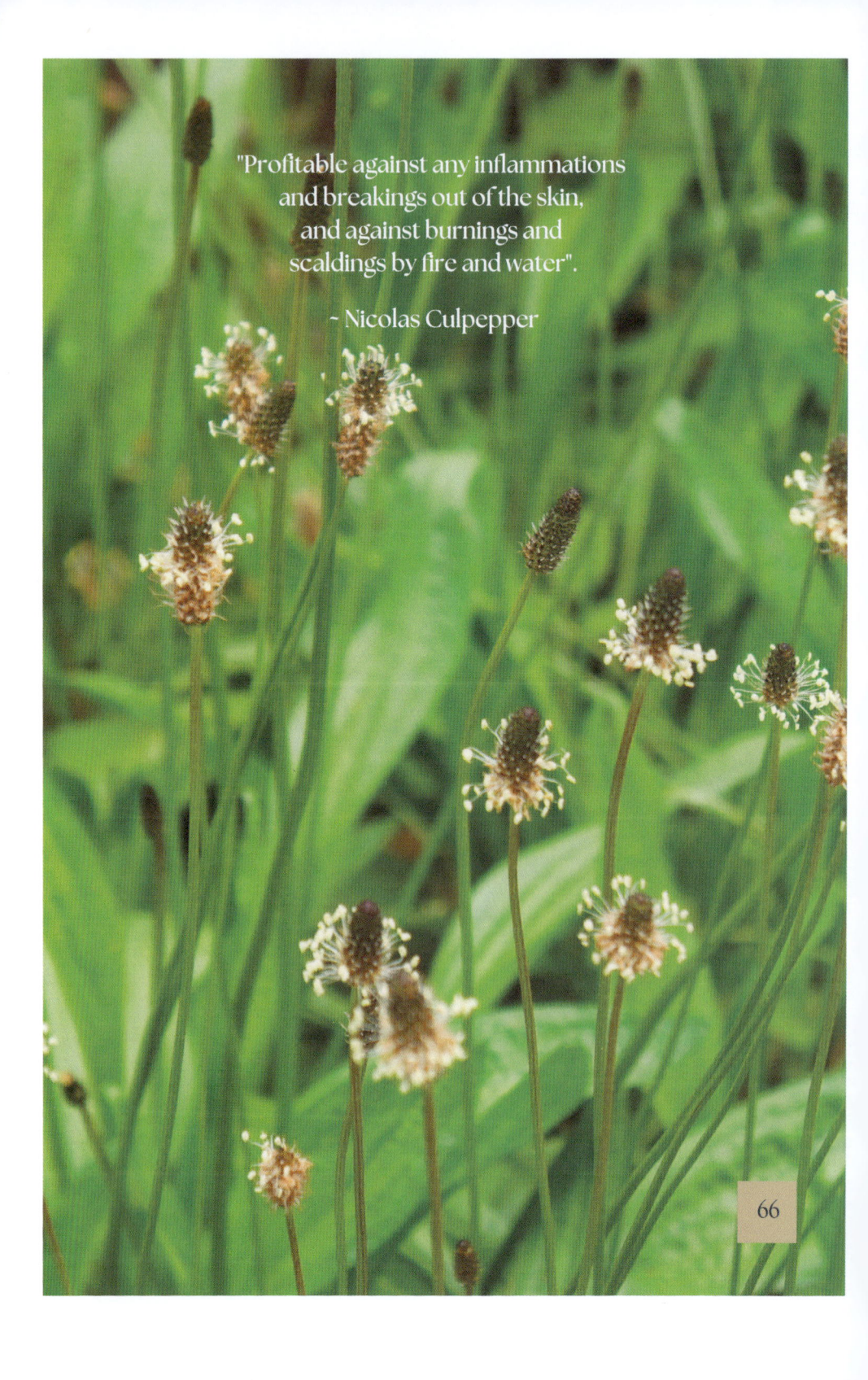

"Profitable against any inflammations
and breakings out of the skin,
and against burnings and
scaldings by fire and water".

~ Nicolas Culpepper

♂HAWTHORN

Latin Name: *Crataegus monogyra and oxycanthoides*

Family Name: Rosaceae family (Strawberry, raspberry, apple, rose)

Other Names:
Fairy tree, May thorn,
White thorn, Thorn apple
Quick thorn, and Pixie pears

Parts Used: flowering tops, leaves, and berries

Habitat: Hawthorn is a hedgerow herb common throughout Great Britain and across Europe.

Identification: large and thorny shrub that grows up to 10 metres tall. Hawthorn has 3-5 lobed leaves with white or pink clusters of flowers. The red fruits or haws come in the Autumn.

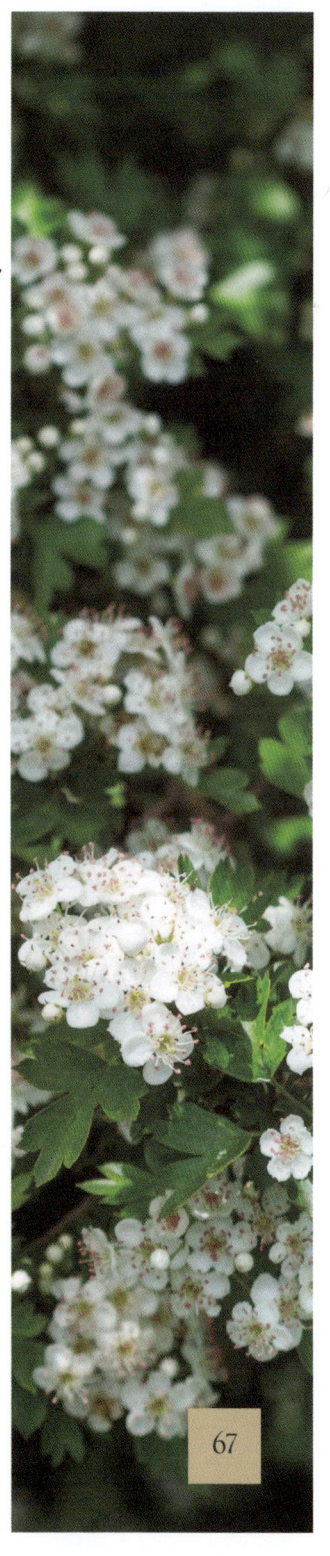

History & Folklore

An amazing heart tonic known about since antiquity. Referred to by Dioscorides, Greek herbalist of 100 AD as Crataegus 'oxuakantha'. The botanical name Crataegus oxyacantha comes from the Greek 'kratos' meaning hardness and 'oxus' meaning sharp and 'akantha' meaning thorn. The latin word Crataegus means 'strong' and 'sharp'.

In old English it was known as 'bread and cheese' as poor village children would eat the leaves and unopened flower heads on their way to and from school for extra nutrition.

Believed to be a meeting place of the faeries, it is considered bad luck to chop down a hawthorn.

Interestingly, hawthorn's main pollinator is the fly, the spiritual symbolism of which means to have compassion for the offensive in life.

History & Folklore

Britain's most sacred hawthorn is said to be in Glastonbury. It is believed that on visiting the Isle of Avalon in Somerset, Joseph of Arimathea rested on "weary-all hill", now called "worral hill". It is here that he stuck his staff he brought from Palastine into the ground and it is from this that the hawthorn tree grew. This tree is considered sacred and believed to blossom on Christmas day.

Another Christian reference to hawthorn comes from the 'crown of thorns' worn by Jesus on the crucifixion which was believed to be made of hawthorns.

A protective tree, used as boundary hedging for millennia. A farmer who plants, respects and protects hawthorn will have fertile soil. Another reason we ask for permission before harvesting.

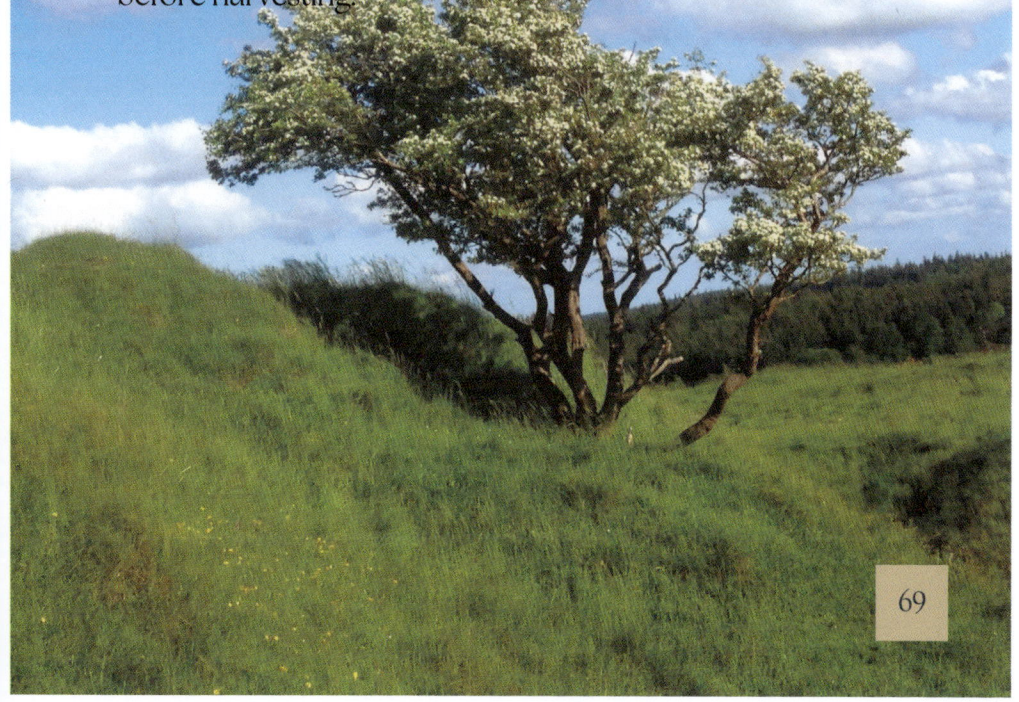

Healing Properties

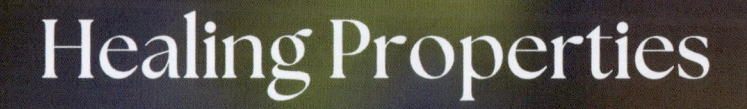

Antioxidant

Anti-inflammatory

Vasodilator

Antispasmodic

Anti-sclerotic

Cardiac tonic

Anti-arrhythmic

Trophorestorative

Anti-hypotensive

Adaptogenic

Medicinal Uses

High blood pressure

Improves circulation

Arrhythmia

Dizziness

Palpitations

Anxiety

Diarrhoea

Over-work

Post-childbirth

Raynaud's phenomenon

Sportmans endurance

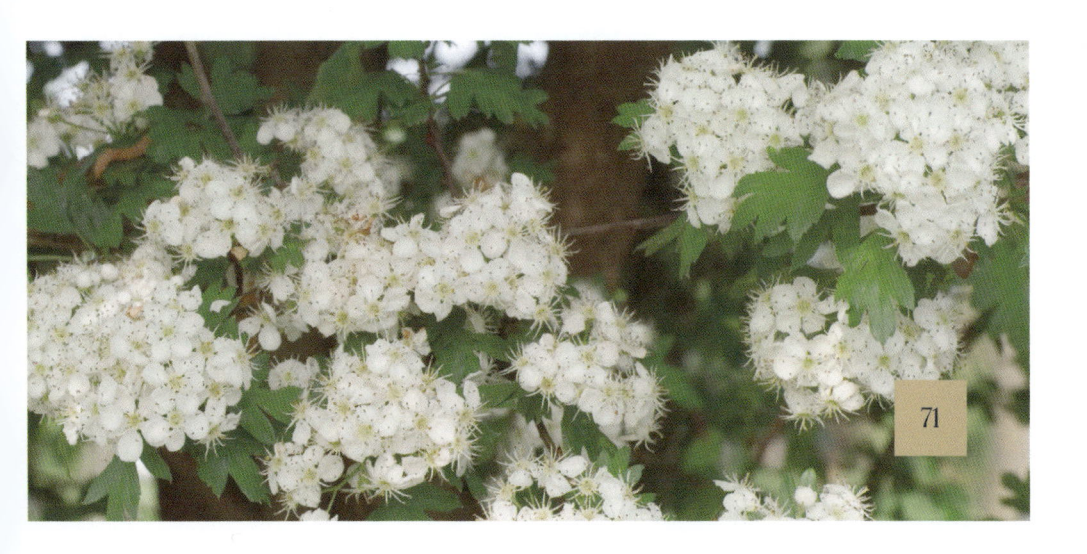

Recipes With Hawthorn

SYRUP

1/2-1 cup of fresh flowers
3-4 tablespoons of water
1/4- 1/2 cup of sugar (we use coconut sugar)

Remove the petals from their stems and green bracts. This can take some time. Add a layer of blossom into a clean jar. Add a layer of sugar on top. Add another layer of blossom. Add another layer of sugar on top of the blossom. Continue layering the sugar and blossoms until you have use all of your sugar and blossoms.

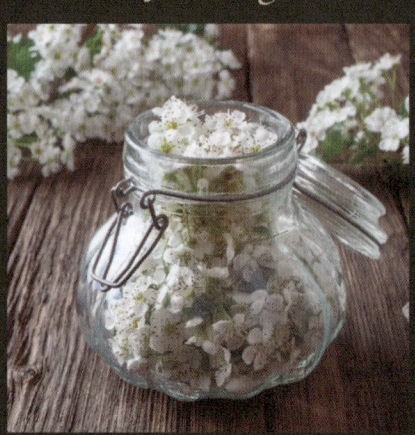

Add 3-4 tablespoons of water (i use hawthorn tea for extra loveliness) to the sugar and fresh/blossom mix. Place a muslin cloth over your jar.

Place the jar into a saucepan and add water around the jar until it is about two thirds up the side of the jar. Ensure the water around the jar does not go dry, so keep topping it up if need be. Heat on a low heat for about an hour and until the sugar has dissolved.

Take the jar out of the saucepan to cool. Screw on the lid and sit overnight. In the morning, strain the flower blossom through a muslin cloth and decant into a clean jar.

This will keep for 2-3 months

Recipes With Hawthorn

HAWTHORN BLOSSOM HONEY

1/2-1 cup of fresh flowers
3-4 tablespoons of water
1/4- 1/2 cup of sugar (we use coconut sugar)

Repeat as per the syrup recipe omitting the sugar layers for honey

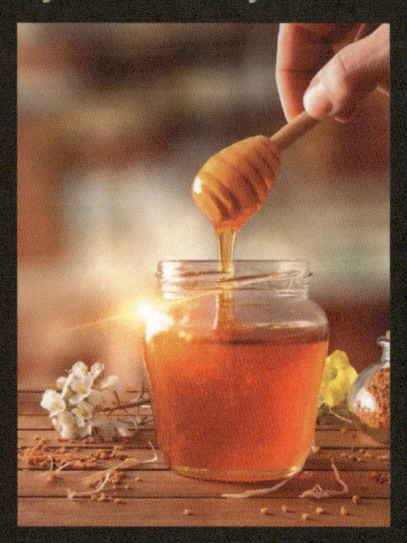

BREAD AND CHEESE

Add the unopened flower buds and young leaves to salads or eat them raw.

SALAD

Fresh young hawthorn leaves (you can use older leaves at different times of year, they are just crunchier and less crisp that the fresh Spring leaves)
Fresh unopened flowers

Wash the young leaves and flower buds.
Prepare your salad, such as spinach, lettuces, rocket, endive, and cucumber. Be creative here and make it delicious and nutritious.

Sprinkle over your salad with the fresh leaves and unopened flower buds. Drizzle with olive oil. Squeeze fresh lemon juice onto your salad. Enjoy your meal.

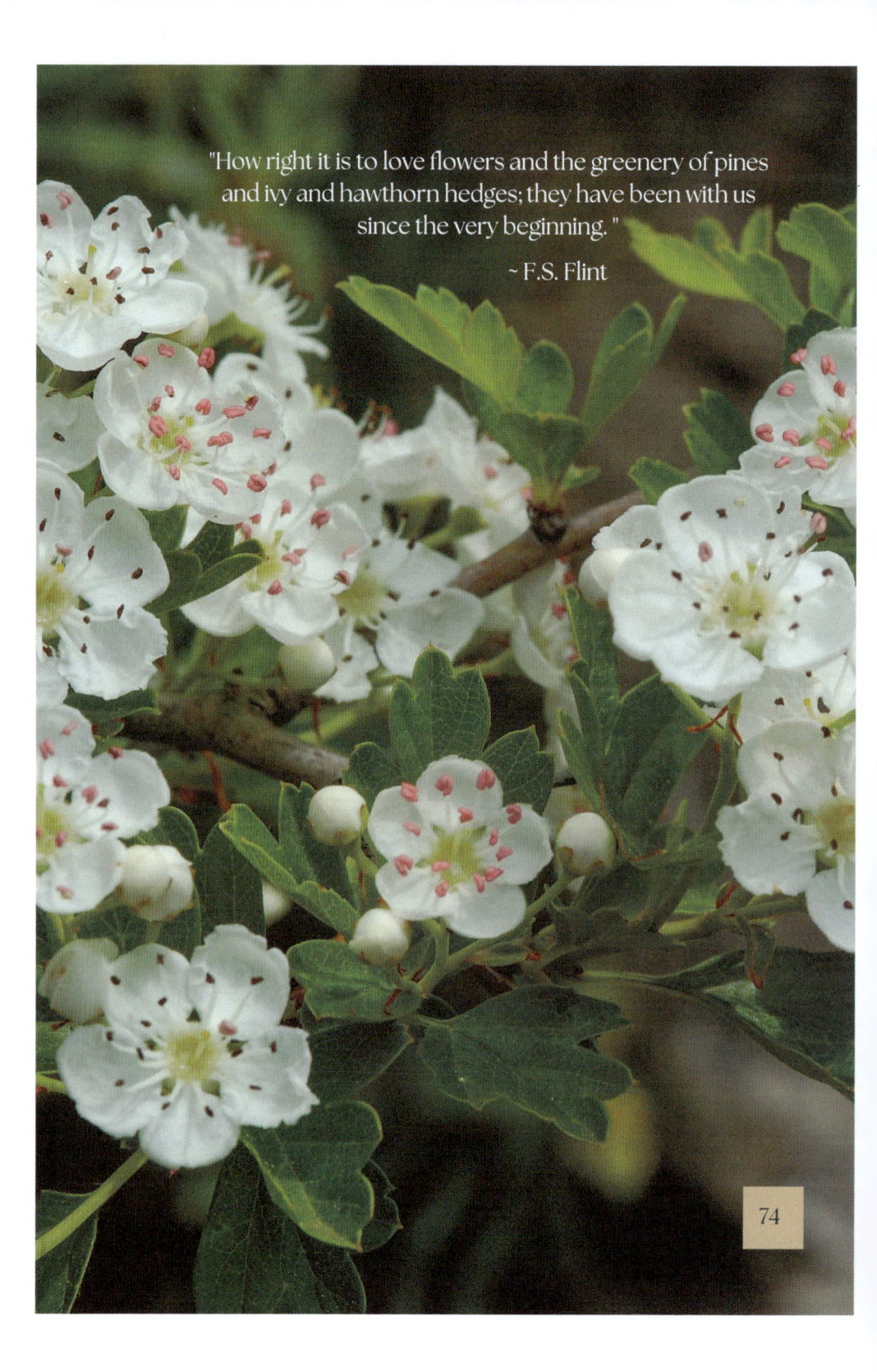

"How right it is to love flowers and the greenery of pines and ivy and hawthorn hedges; they have been with us since the very beginning."

~ F.S. Flint

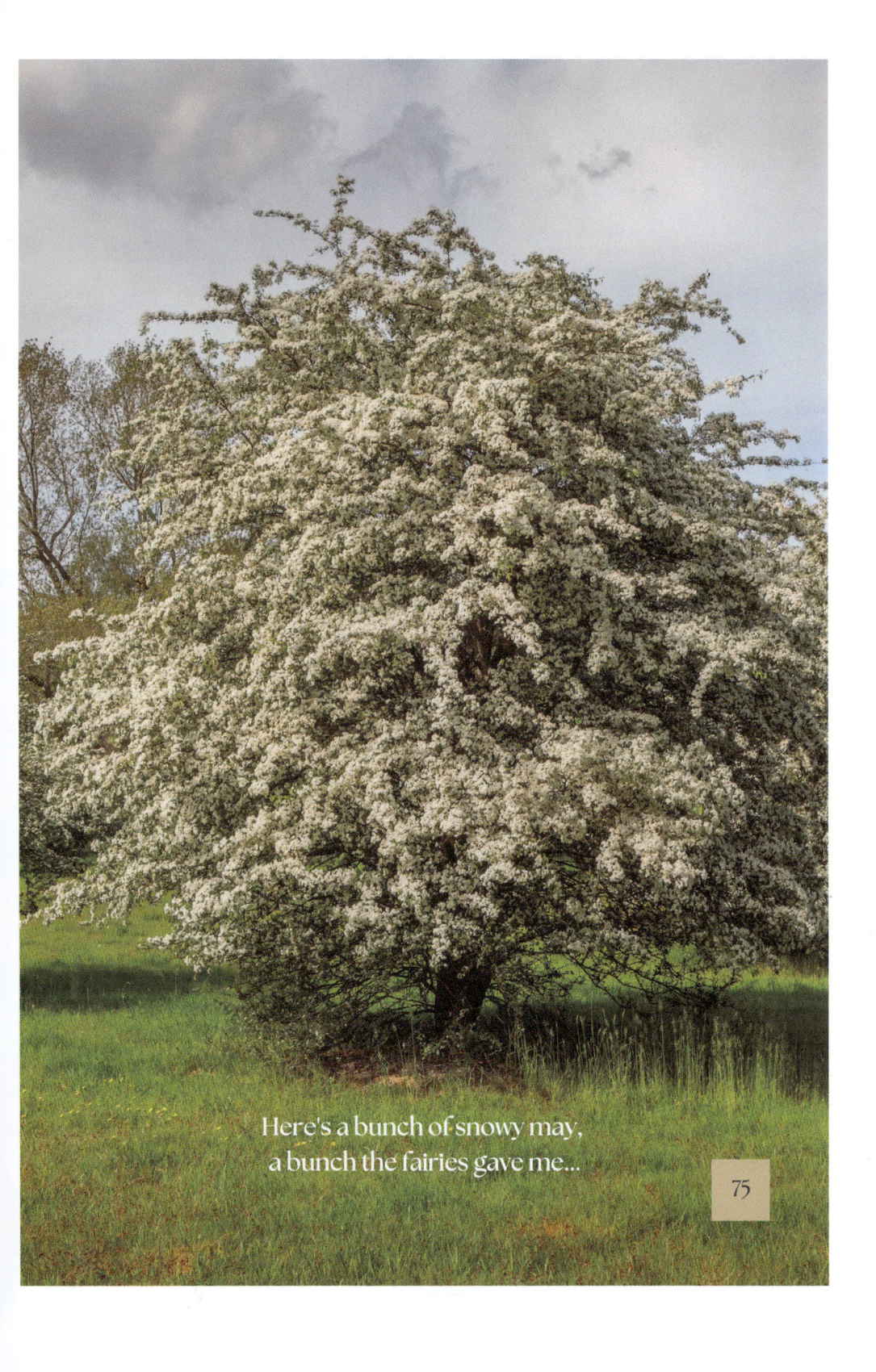

Here's a bunch of snowy may,
a bunch the fairies gave me...

♂ NETTLE

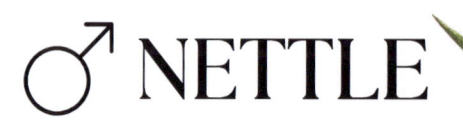

Latin Name: *Urtica dioica*

Family Name:
Urticaceae family
(Pellitory, asthma weed, dead nettle)

Other Names:
stinging nettle,
devils leaf

Parts Used: whole herb, leaves, roots, flowering tops and seeds

Habitat: waste and cultivated ground, wet woodland, everywhere

Identification:
Heart shaped toothy coarse leaves with fine stinging hairs and thin catkins of seeds.

History & Folklore

Nettle seeds were found on Roman remains from 200 years ago. However their history goes back as long as man's. Nettle was a most important plant for our ancestors, providing nutrition, clothing and potent medicine.

As Neolithic tribes cleared woods for their settlements, nettles would spring up everywhere and were used to provide fibre for string, fishing nets and cloth.
Nettle fibre is incredibly strong.

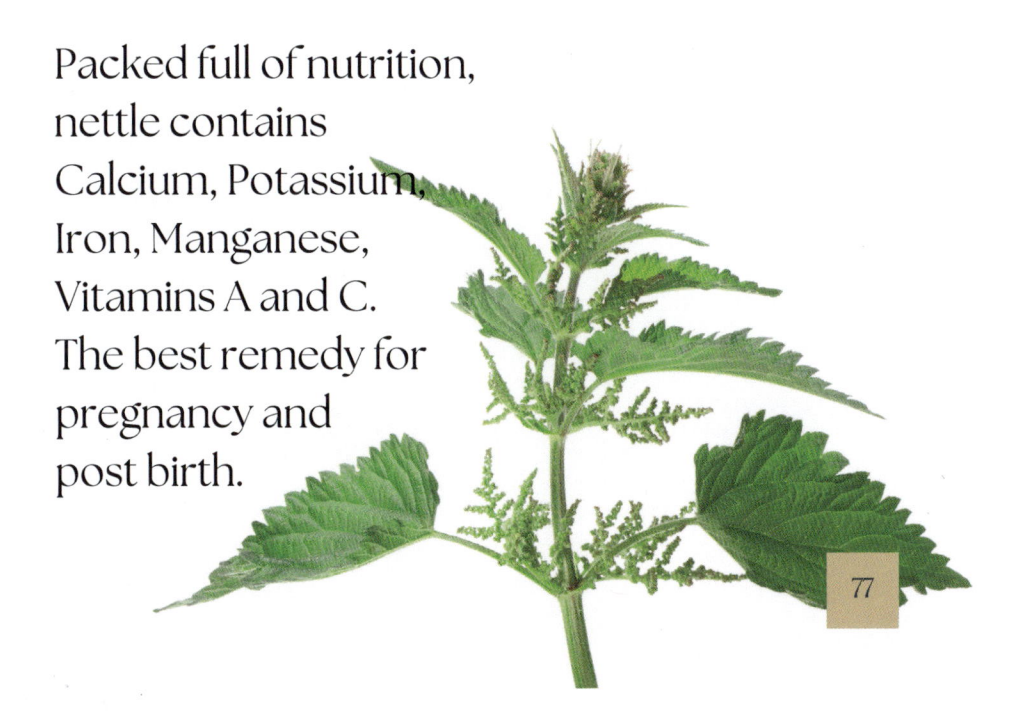

Packed full of nutrition, nettle contains Calcium, Potassium, Iron, Manganese, Vitamins A and C.
The best remedy for pregnancy and post birth.

History & Folklore

In the olden times nettle was associated with the God Thor. In order to win his favour, travellers would throw big bunches of nettle on to the fire as a worship to Thor, so that he would bless their journey and keep the lightning at bay.

Nettle is a symbol of protection.

A traditional herbal remedy is urtication which is the flogging of the limbs with nettles to aid arthritis and rheumatism.

Therapeutic Use

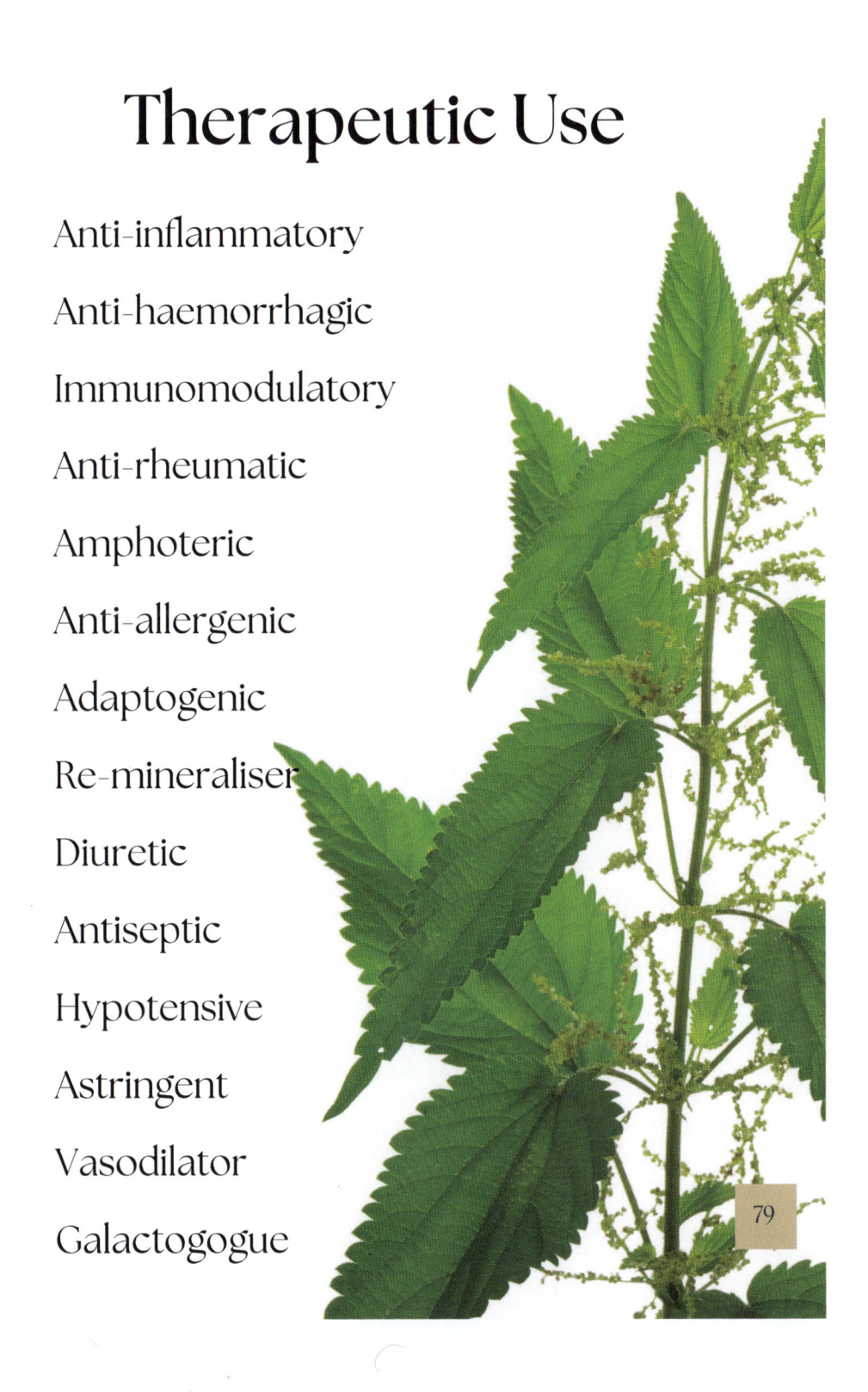

Anti-inflammatory

Anti-haemorrhagic

Immunomodulatory

Anti-rheumatic

Amphoteric

Anti-allergenic

Adaptogenic

Re-mineraliser

Diuretic

Antiseptic

Hypotensive

Astringent

Vasodilator

Galactogogue

Medicinal Uses

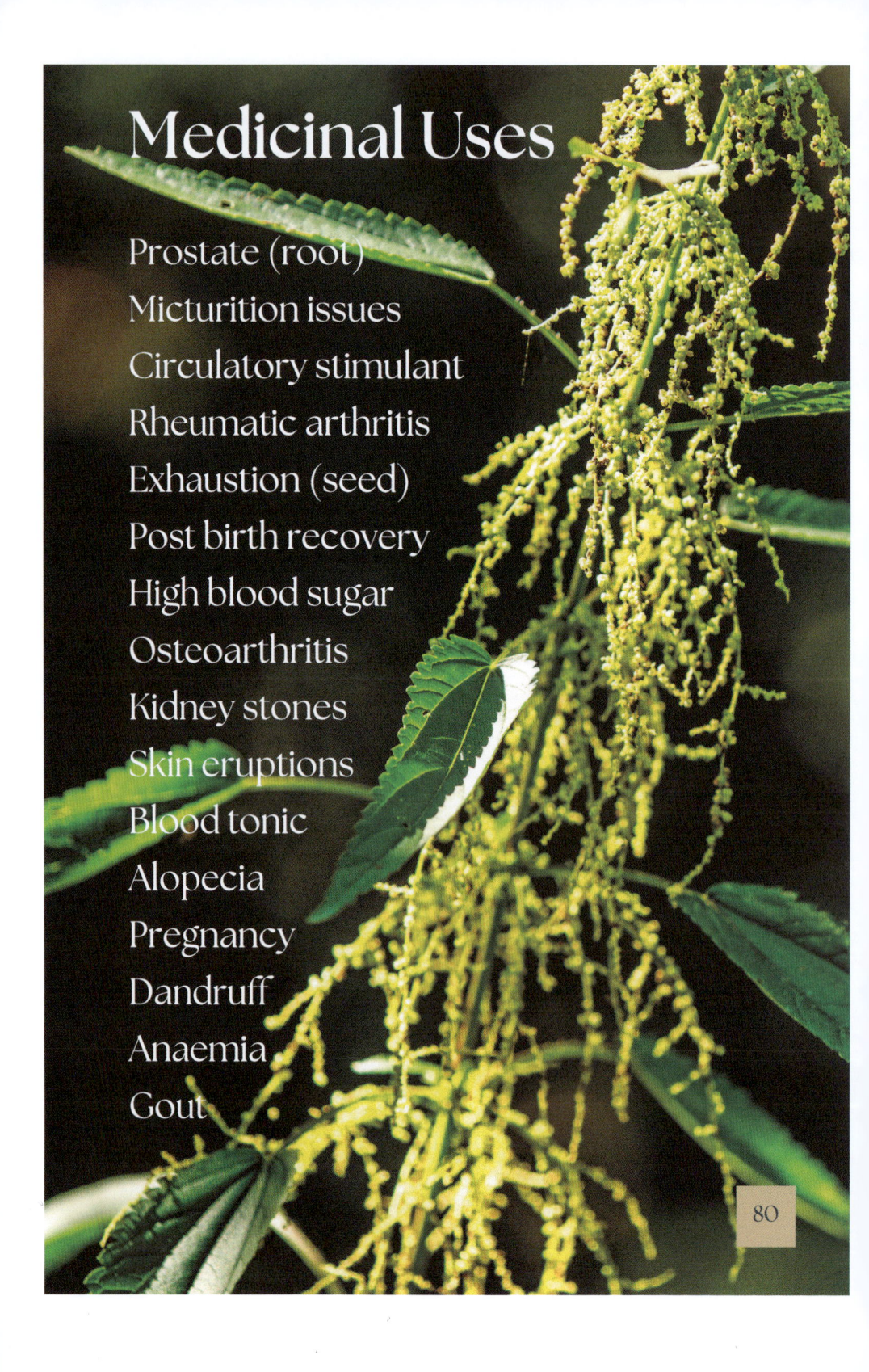

Prostate (root)
Micturition issues
Circulatory stimulant
Rheumatic arthritis
Exhaustion (seed)
Post birth recovery
High blood sugar
Osteoarthritis
Kidney stones
Skin eruptions
Blood tonic
Alopecia
Pregnancy
Dandruff
Anaemia
Gout

Recipes With Nettle

NETTLE SOUP

2x Large Bowls of Nettle tops
2x onion or shallots chopped
25gm butter/vegan alternative
1Tblsp olive oil
2x medium potatoes peeled
2 sticks of celery chopped
Salt & pepper seasoning
Bay leaf
Sprig of thyme
4x cups of stock/water
3 Tbls cream (if desired)

Blanch nettles in boiling water for 2 minutes. Remove and place in cold water and drain.

In a pan, heat butter and olive oil, add onion/shallots and celery. Cook to soften for 5x minutes. Add chopped potato, stock, bay, thyme and pinch of salt. Simmer for 5 minutes

Chop cooked nettles, add 4 cups to a pan with enough water to cover. Simmer for 15-20 minutes until potatoes cooked. Remove herbs, puree, add lemon juice, black pepper and stir cream in to serve.

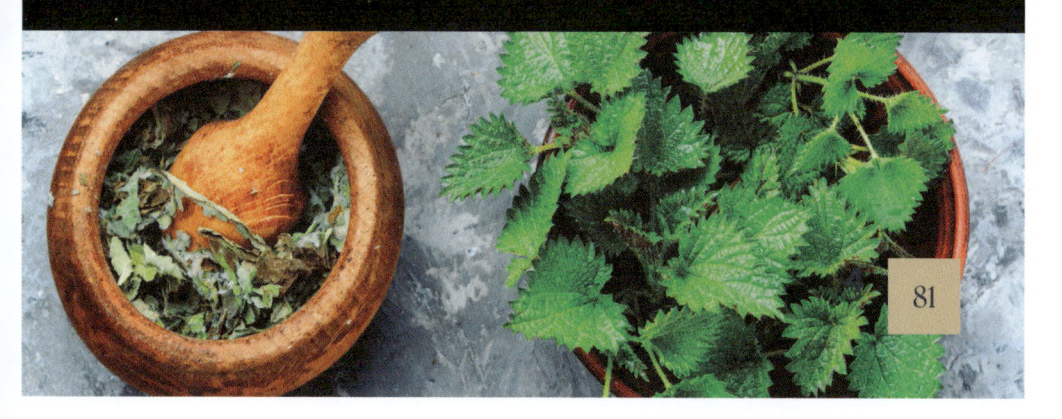

Recipes With Nettle

JUICE
Juice nettles as part of a seasonal Spring cleanse detoxification. The deep chlorophyll green colour is pure superfood.

VEGETABLE
Wilt washed nettle leaves in a pan with a knob of butter or olive oil and a clove of garlic or leaves of wild garlic. Makes a lovely side dish and can be added to omelettes, pasta or just on its own.

FACIAL STEAM
Fill a basin or bowl with hot water, submerge a handful of nettle tops. Place face above but not touching the water, cover head with towel. an steam. Helps eczema. and complexion.

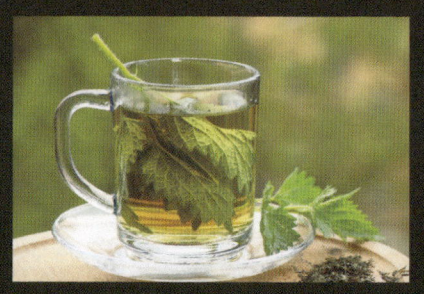

TEA
An amazingly healthy drink, add a few sprigs of fresh washed leaves to a pot of hot water. Great combined with fresh mint. Energising.

COMPOST
Sit cut nettles in a covered bucket of rainwater, leave for 2-4 weeks. Use it to fertilise the garden. Very smelly but nutritious.

HAIR TONIC
Make as tea, cool and use as final rinse in the shower.

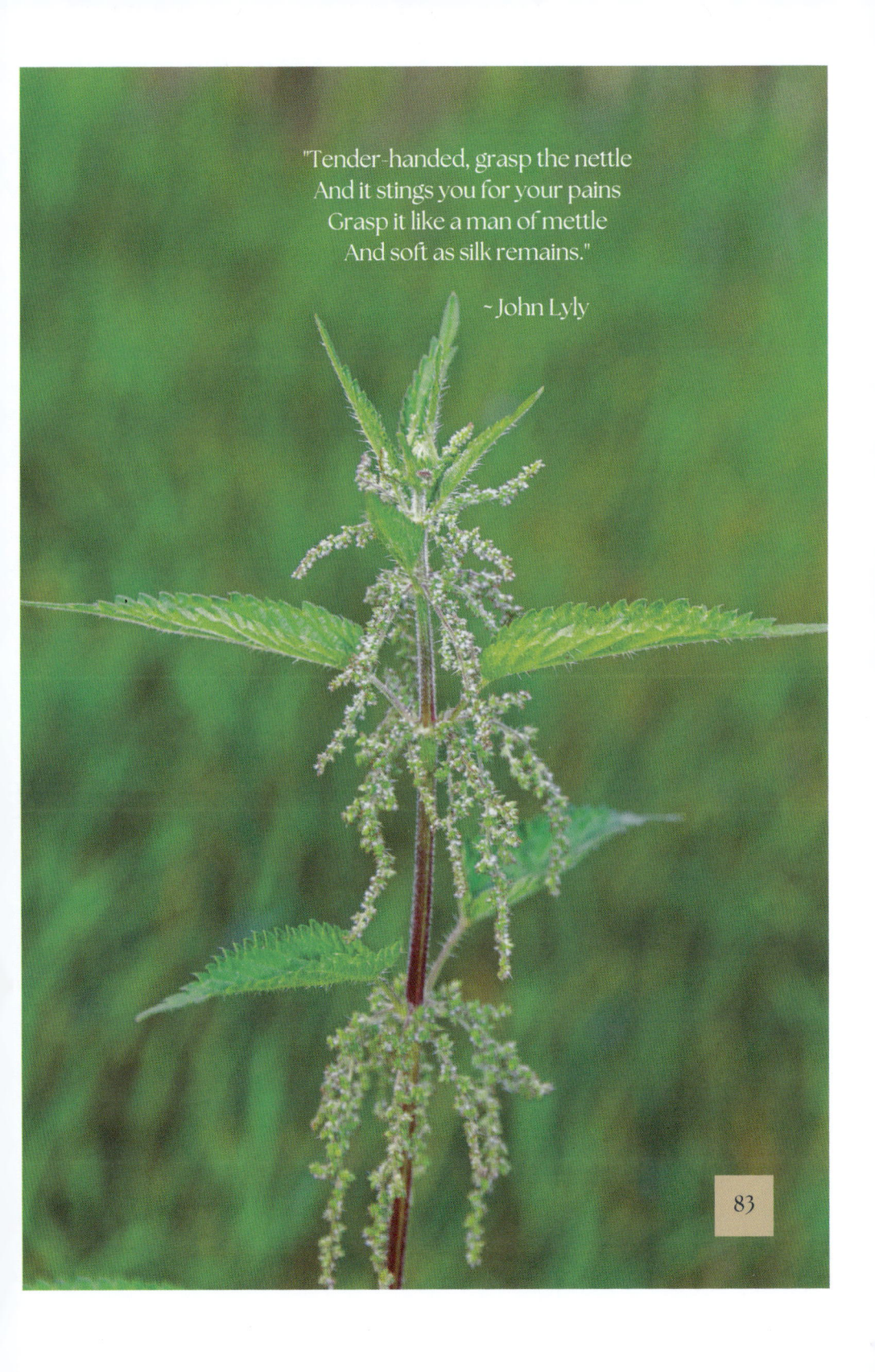

"Tender-handed, grasp the nettle
And it stings you for your pains
Grasp it like a man of mettle
And soft as silk remains."

~ John Lyly

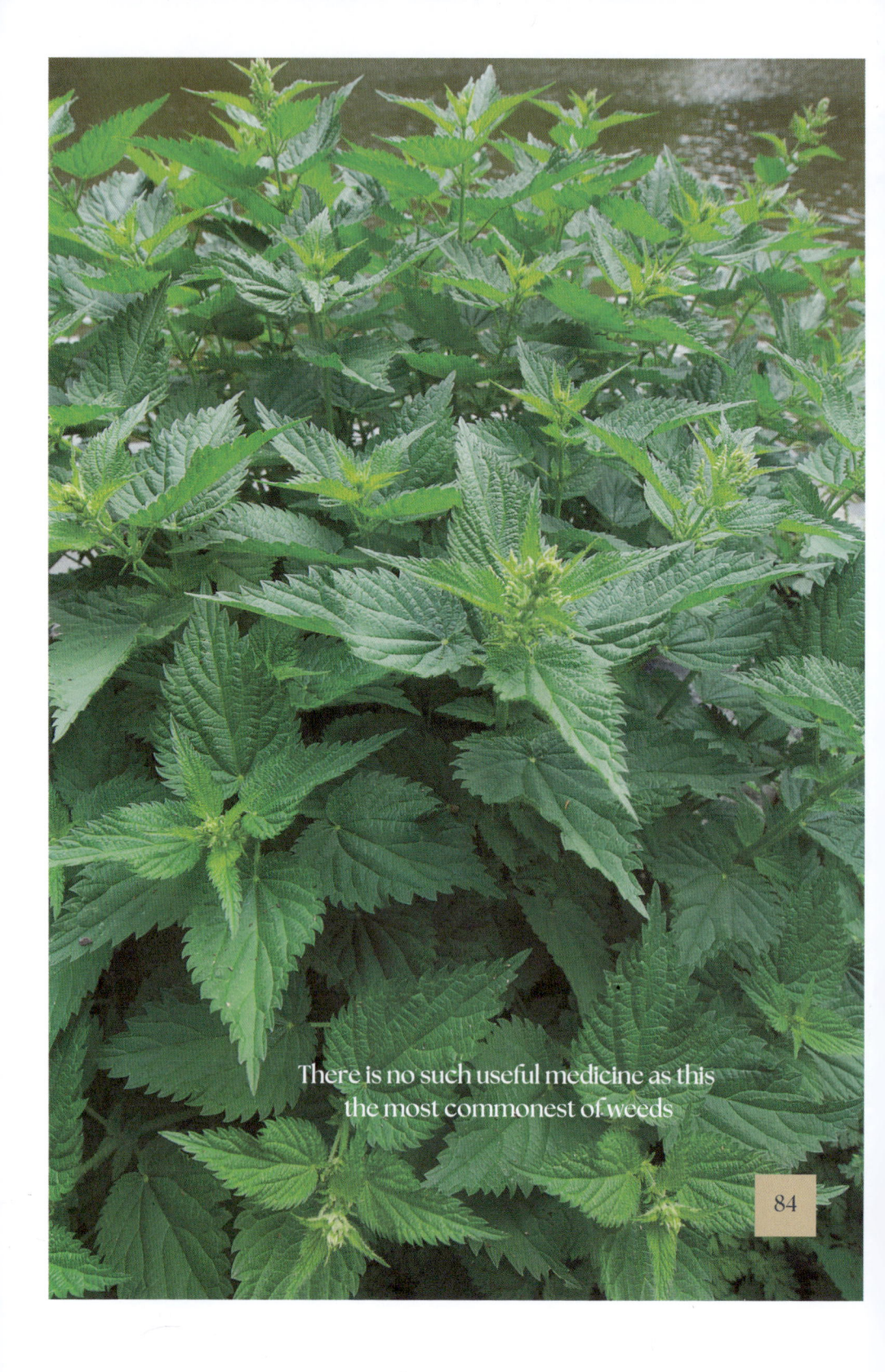

There is no such useful medicine as this
the most commonest of weeds

Planetary Symbols

The Ancient Greeks believed the planets had dominion over plants, stones, colours, the bodily organs, the nature of disease and even the days of the week. They believed that planetary astrology affected everything:

'As above, so below.'

☽ **Moon** herbs are light coloured preferring moist environments. Cool and moist. The moon rules over the eyesight along with the sun. Culpepper suggested the moon rules over 'the left eye of man, and the right eye of woman'. The moon governs the waters of the body, intestines, brain along with the sun), hormones and amniotic fluids.

☉ **Sun** herbs are bright, yellow and need full sun. The sun rules over the heart but also the brain (predominantly male) and the eyes. Hot and dry. Associated with our sense of sight, our spirit, vital energy and life force.

Planetary Symbols

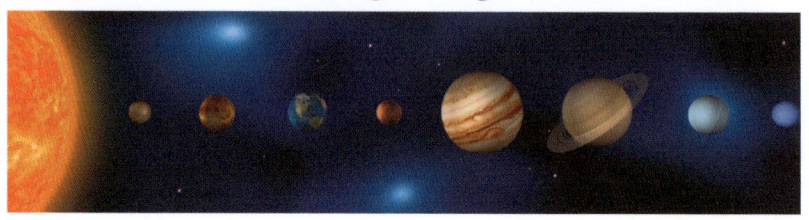

♀ **Venus** herbs are soft and pleasing to the senses and nourishing to their environment. Warm and moist in nature they have an affinity with our sense of touch or feeling. Ruler of the kidneys, throat, skin, sperm and ovaries.

♂ **Mars** herbs are thorny, have barbs or sting Their actions are stimulating and defensive in nature. Hot and dry constitutions. Spicy and firey. Rash, war-like, mars literally gets things done. Associated with the gallbladder, kidney and gall bladder stones, fevers and fistulas.

Our ancestors understood that herbs gathered under a particular planetary alignment would be helpful for a certain condition or constitution. Paracelsus and later Culpepper related these to the four humours or states of a persons health/constitutions: Sanguine, Choleric, Melancholy and Phlegmatic which relate to the four elements Air, Fire, Earth and Water.

GLOSSARY

ADAPTOGENIC	Increases resistance to stress
ALTERATIVE	Improves detoxification, & blood
AMPHORETIC	Adjusts the flow of breast milk
ANALGESIC	Pain killer
ANTI-HAEMORRHAGIC	Stops bleeding
ANTIHISTAMINE	Reduces allergic reaction
ANTIOXIDANT	Prevent damage from free radicals
ANTIPRURITIC	Stops itching
ANTIRHEUMATIC	Prevents or relieves rheumatism
ANTISPASMODIC	Reduces muscle contractions
APERIENT	Relieves constipation
ASTRINGENT	Drying, drawing, shrinking action
CHOLAGOGUE	Promotes discharge of bile
DEMULCENT	Relieves irritation & inflammation
DEPURITIVE	Purifying and detoxifying
DETOXIFICATION	Cleansing, blood purifying
EMMOLIENT	Soften, soothes, moistens lesions
FEBRIFUGE	Reduces fever
GALACTAGOGUE	Increases breast milk production
HEPATOPROTECTIVE	Prevents damage to the liver
HYPOGLYCAEMIC	Increase insulin secretion
HYPOTENSIVE	Reduces blood pressure
IMMUNOMODULATORY	Balances immune system activity
MICTURITION	Expels urine from the body
MUCILAGINOS	Mucous like substance
REFRIGERANT	Cooling, soothing irritation
TONIC	Builds, strengthens and nourishes
VASODILATOR	Dilates, widens blood vessels. Heals wounds
VULNERARY	

Your Health is in Your Hands

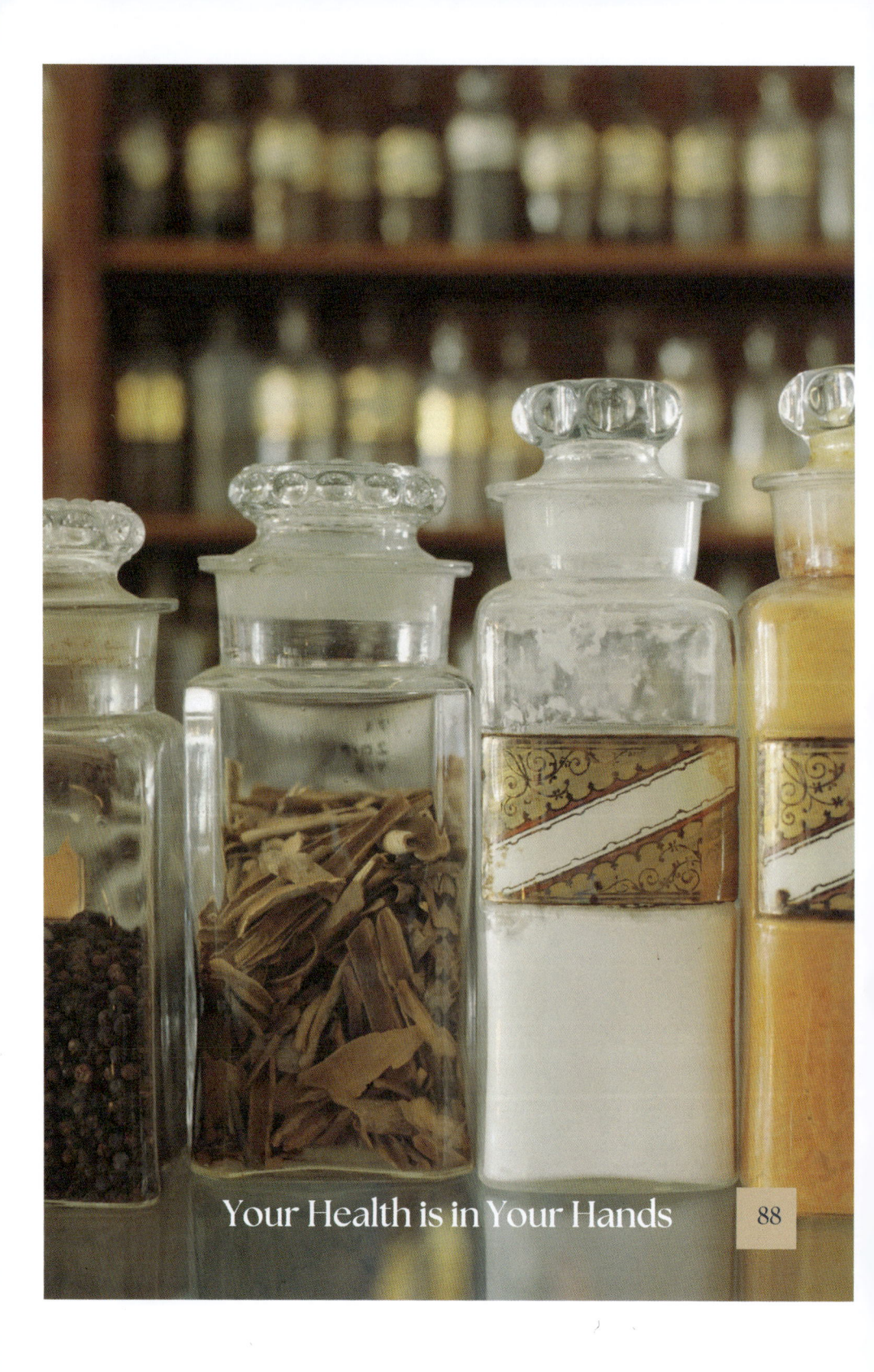

About the Author

Caroline is a fully qualified herbalist, naturopath, nutrition consultant but more than that she is an intuitive healer, one who hears the whispers of the plants called upon to heal the individuals she sees in her clinic.

She inherited a deep connection to the land and the healing plant kingdom from her ancestry. In her youth, Caroline set up a successful herbal garden and farmers markets in Cyprus. Here she learned from the village elders and was awarded for her work with local culture, sustainability and the environment.

Her theoretical knowledge, extensive experience in clinic and practical application learned by working so closely with the plants makes her one of life's leading lights whose words truly come from a depth of understanding, integrity and wisdom.

For more information:
youtube caroline evans herbalist
www.heavenonearthherbals.com

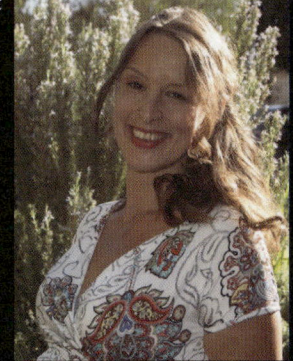

About the Author

Caroline delivered her first online course in 2022 which was a great success and now has a list of upcoming courses as well as a yearly membership program. If you would like to take part in one of her live workshops and courses or to join the monthly 'Build your Herbal Medicine Chest' where we build your herbal and health knowledge on a month by month basis.

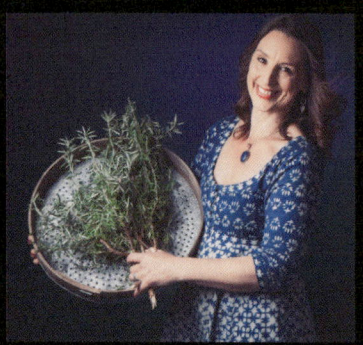

www.heavenonearthherbals.com

Testimonials from the recent course:

"Caroline is truly a master herbalist, nutritionist and naturopath.. and a beautiful generous soul. This week was packed full of useful information, beautifully presented visually, and with an eye to empowering her students in the realm of wise self-care, so crucial in these turbulent times. Just a real treat! If you have a chance to attend one of her courses, or to work with her individually, don't hesitate."   ~ Melanie Reinhart

"The course, 'Boost your immune system in 5 days', was very informative and highly accessible. Caroline delivers the information clearly, enthusiastically and, importantly, in a non-judgemental manner. She generously shares her knowledge and encourages and inspires you to discover more about your body's amazing capacities and to have a go at making simple home remedies for common ailments."   ~ Alison Kavannagh

Printed in Great Britain
by Amazon